'This is by far one of the most engaging and compelling discussions on nursing ethics to be published this century. At last we have a book that comprehensively and convincingly captures the "moral project" of nursing and the unique moral quandaries that nurses face when trying to fulfil their professional obligations to provide individualised nursing care in contexts increasingly constrained by economic considerations and various resource restraints. This book not only captures the specific moral quandaries nurses face when trying to balance the competing needs of patients for nursing care, but provides a new ethical framework for addressing these quandaries'.

Professor Megan-Jane Johnstone, School of Nursing and Midwifery,
Deakin University, Geelong, Australia

Partiality and Justice in Nursing Care

Partiality and Justice in Nursing Care examines the conflicting normative claims of partiality and impartiality in nursing care, looking in depth at how to reconcile reasonable concerns for one particular patient with equally important concerns for the maximisation of health-related welfare for all with relevant nursing-care needs, in a resource-limited setting.

Drawing on moral philosophy, this book explores how discussions of partiality and impartiality in moral philosophy can have relevance to the professional context of clinical nursing care as well as in nursing ethics in general. It develops a framework for normative nursing ethics that incorporates a notion of permissible partiality, and specifies which concerns an ethics of nursing care should entail when balancing partialist and impartialist concerns. At the same time, Nordhaug argues that this partiality must also be constrained by both principled and context-sensitive assessments of patients' needs, as well as of the role-relative deontological restriction of minimising harm, something that could be mitigated by institutional and organisational arrangements.

This thought-provoking volume is an important contribution to nursing ethics and philosophy.

Marita Nordhaug is Associate Professor at Oslo and Akershus University College of Applied Sciences, Faculty of Health Sciences, Norway. She has a professional background as a nurse (RN), and holds a Master's Degree in Nursing Science, and a Ph.D. in the Study of Professions. Nordhaug has also been an associate Ph.D. student in the Ethics Programme, University of Oslo, Norway.

Routledge Key Themes in Health and Society

https://www.routledge.com/Routledge-Key-Themes-in-Health-and-Society/book-series/RKTHS

Available titles include:

The Story of Nursing in British Mental Hospitals
Echoes from the corridors
Niall McCrae and Peter Nolan

Living with Mental Disorder
Insights from qualitative research
Jacqueline Corcoran

A New Ethic of 'Older'
Subjectivity, Surgery and Self-stylization
Bridget Garnham

Social Theory and Nursing
Edited by Martin Lipscomb

Older Citizens and End-of-Life Care
Social work practice strategies for adults in later life
Malcolm Payne

Digital Technologies and Generational Identity
ICT Usage Across the Life Course
Sakari Taipale, Terhi-Anna Wilksa and Chris Gilleard

Partiality and Justice in Nursing Care
Marita Nordhaug

Forthcoming titles include:

Identity, Ageing and Cultural Adaptation
Understanding longevity in crossdisciplinary perspective
Simon Biggs

Partiality and Justice in Nursing Care

Marita Nordhaug

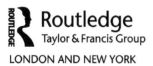

Routledge
Taylor & Francis Group

LONDON AND NEW YORK

First published 2018 by Routledge

2 Park Square, Milton Park, Abingdon, Oxfordshire OX14 4RN

52 Vanderbilt Avenue, New York, NY 10017

Routledge is an imprint of the Taylor & Francis Group, an informa business

First issued in paperback 2019

British Library Cataloguing in Publication Data
A catalogue record for this book is available from the British Library

Library of Congress Cataloging in Publication Data
Names: Nordhaug, Marita, author.
Title: Partiality and justice in nursing care / Marita Nordhaug.
Description: Milton Park, Abingdon, Oxon ; New York, NY : Routledge, 2017. | Includes bibliographical references and index.
Identifiers: LCCN 2017005825 | ISBN 9780415792813 (hbk) | ISBN 9781315211381 (ebk)
Subjects: LCSH: Nursing ethics.
Classification: LCC RT85 .N67 2017 | DDC 174.2/9073--dc23
LC record available at https://lccn.loc.gov/2017005825

ISBN: 978-0-415-79281-3 (hbk)
ISBN: 978-0-367-22450-9 (pbk)

Typeset in Times New Roman
by Taylor & Francis Books

Contents

Preface

'Please let me know when you feel ready for a walk', the nurse said to me. It was the evening shift on Friday, and it was hectic in the ward. I was in a hospital bed, feeling quite well, but after having surgery the previous day I was unable to get out of bed without assistance. I knew this nurse was busy. I knew because my door was open. I heard a patient crying in pain, I heard the alarm bells, I saw physicians and nurses rushing in the corridors, I saw a patient return from the postoperative unit. Besides, as a nurse myself I knew that an evening shift on weekends means less personnel but not less to do. Still, this nurse came to me, smiling and offering to take a walk with me in the corridor. 'I would love to. But you are busy. Besides, I have already been out of bed twice today', I replied. 'That's good', she replied. 'But taking you for a walk is just as important a task for me just as anything else this evening. So just let me know when you're in less pain and feel ready for a walk.'

This event took place a few years ago, and to me this nurse's attitude and understanding of responsibility is an example worthy of imitation. One might read this scenario as a nurse simply doing her job. This nurse was my keeper. But she was also the keeper for other patients, and caring for the needs of many often entails potential conflicts around the distribution of time and attention. Nurses are patients' keepers. But when faced with multiple and rival moral concerns, and when there is no solution free of costs, *which* patient's keeper should I be? This book studies the conflicting normative claims of partiality and impartiality in nursing care, and aims to establish a sound argument for permissible partiality in nursing care.

The book is a revised edition of my Ph.D. thesis titled *Which Patient's Keeper? Partiality and Justice in Nursing Care* from the Centre for the Study of Professions, Oslo and Akershus University College of Applied Sciences. Permission for republishing has been granted. Given the central role that the concept of need has for the arguments and discussions concerning partiality and justice in nursing care, a new chapter devoted to an analysis of the need concept was produced and included in this book. Apart from Chapter 3, which addresses this subject, the book comprises a lightly revised version of the original manuscript.

Acknowledgements

The squirrel that you kill in jest, dies in earnest. This line, stemming from Henry David Thoreau, crossed my mind many years ago. And it has stayed there. To me it signifies that what sometimes, or by someone, is considered insignificant, is of most significant value for someone else. It also accentuates awareness for the fact that even a decision that seems minor, might have deep impact and severe consequences for the life and dignity of someone else, and even for the one making the choice. In some sense, this is what this book is about. At least, it represents my motivational force for writing it.

I would like to thank everyone who has supported me throughout this work. During these years there have been more people than I can now list, but still some whom I will acknowledge in particular. I owe my deepest gratitude to Per Nortvedt and Jan Helge Solbakk at the Center for Medical Ethics, University of Oslo. Per, I owe you heartfelt thanks for being a fabulous adviser, and the source of professional inspiration you have been for me for many years, and still are. Jan Helge, I am forever thankful for your faith in me. The original thesis was funded by the Centre for the Study of Professions (SPS), Oslo and Akershus University College of Applied Sciences (HiOA). I am very grateful for having been a part of this stimulating academic environment. In particular, I wish to thank Oddgeir Osland, Director of SPS, for support, and for giving me the opportunity to work with the chapter on the need concept. I wish to express great appreciation to the academic community at the Ethics Program, University of Oslo, of which I had the privilege of being an associated Ph.D. student. Thanks also to the members of the seminar of care ethics at the Centre for Medical Ethics, University of Oslo, for inspiring discussions on the ethics of care.

I am also particularly thankful to Per Nortvedt, Harald Grimen, Anders Molander, Edmund Henden, and Jan Helge Solbakk for providing invaluable feedback on drafts of the original thesis, as well as to the expert assessment committee of the original thesis, Nils Gilje, Steven Edwards, and Kristine Bærøe, for a thorough and constructive review. Thanks to my colleagues at the Department of Nursing and Health Promotion, HiOA, campus Kjeller, for your support and motivational boosts.

Finally, I want to express my deepest thanks to my friends and family for your care, patience and support.

Marita Nordhaug
Eidsvoll, January 2017

Introduction

Due to their social terms of reference, nurses should distribute their available time according to impartial perspectives and prescriptions. For instance, they should give due consideration to the needs of patients according to criteria of severity and urgency. Being a patient's caretaker is, however, not only about assessing the severity and urgency of a patient's needs for care and medical treatment. Indeed, it is also about ensuring that particular patients receive adequate[1] and individualised nursing care. But the ability to reconcile the concern for treating the individual patient properly with the equal concern of tending to all patients according to their health care needs has become a pressing issue for nurses. As a result, conflicting moral claims impinge upon the daily practices of nurses. This dualism also challenges our double set of expectations and assumptions about health care services funded by public money. As Søren Holm puts it,

> Most of us have two strong intuitions (or sets of intuitions) in relation to fairness in health care systems that are funded by public money, whether through taxation or compulsory insurance. The first intuition is that such a system has to treat patients (or other users) fairly, equitably, impartially, justly, and without discrimination. [...] The second intuition is that doctors, nurses and other health care professionals are allowed to, and may even in some cases be obligated to give preference to the interests of the particular patients or clients over the interests of other patients or clients of the system.
>
> (Holm, 2011, p. 90)

These are not only intuitions, though. They are also soundly based on regulations, like those codified by the World Medical Association (World Medical Association, 1948/2006, Declaration of Geneva) and the International Council of Nurses (The ICN Code of Ethics for Nurses, 2006). The ability of a nurse to provide requisite attention to the needs of the individual patient is increasingly becoming constrained, thus amplifying a significant normative imbalance between concerns of relational and individual care and concerns of distributive justice. Recent studies about prioritisations in clinical health care indicate that time and ability to meet the professional ethical imperative of individualised care seems to be frequently compromised.[2] For instance, lack of adequate attention to the needs of elderly patients in Norwegian nursing homes and public hospitals is documented. Time for communication, physical activity, nutrition, and the treatment of minor illnesses and 'silent' psychiatric problems, in addition to basic nursing care, are examples of compromised needs (Pedersen et al., 2008). Jeopardised nursing care not only affects older patients, though. For example, studies carried out in Europe and the USA demonstrate that lack of resources such as time and personnel decreases the ability to provide sufficient nursing care to hospitalised patients in general.[3] Any such research finding illustrates a burning ethical problem since the lack of relational care and concern can result in increased suffering for the patient (Pettersen, 2006). The regime of scarcity and the inability of society to meet the health care needs of all its citizens require a system in which health care is distributed according to the values of fairness, impartiality, and justice. The price to pay, however, is that the quality and normative importance of particularised individual care seems to be jeopardised. This makes debates about reasonable forms of partiality in nursing care increasingly important as a way of finding a proper balance between individual care and distributive considerations. The main argument in this book is that nurses, in some situations, are permitted to be partial in order to fulfil their professional commitment of individualised nursing care. It will argued that in some situations partiality towards a particular patient might trump impartial concerns of distributive justice.

The challenge is how the discussion of partiality can be included within the larger domain of nursing ethics. Moral philosophers have for centuries debated the conflicting claims of partiality and impartiality, going back as far as the Aristotelians and the Stoics (Annas, 1993). But with a few exceptions,[4] the debates have not been conducted within the context of professional care, professional roles, and relationships. Though it may be argued that professional ethics is grounded in, or at least shares important features with, our common sense morality where certain forms of partiality can be argued for, professional ethics is generally characterised by a far stronger emphasis on impartial concerns. Within an impartial outlook, judgments about the content and the scope of professional care should be made according to patients' objective as well as subjective needs. And the decisions also have to be balanced according to budgets and the political guidelines for priority setting. This is also why an argument of permissible partiality has implications for the way nursing ethics in general and nurses' responsibilities in particular are understood.

The argument of this book is that partiality can serve and protect the collective good pursued by the nursing profession. The collective good pursued by the nursing profession regards patients' needs for nursing care, i.e. needs concerning patients' health and medical condition.[5] In nursing practice, pursuing the collective good comes about in concrete caring situations where nurses are committed to performing adequate and individualised nursing care. Moreover, partiality in nursing care is aimed at protecting the integrity of both the patient and the nurse. For these reasons it is crucial to clarify in what way partiality can be normatively justified within professional health care ethics in general and nursing ethics in particular. In the ethics literature, partiality is usually understood as showing greater consideration of the needs of some versus the needs others, for reasons generated by valuable relationships. For reasons I return to later in this book, I will, however, propose an argument for partiality that is not *presupposed* merely on the valuing of the professional relationship per se. As an alternative, I attempt to establish an argument for permissible partiality in situations where partiality is necessary for nurses who are committed to performing adequate and individualised nursing care.

As initially stated, one aspect of nursing ethics which highlights the relevance of various forms of partiality is illuminated by looking at the context of clinical health care prioritisations. Priority decisions take place on several levels in the health care system. Bærøe (2009), for instance, describes four levels of decision-making as (1) the superior level of state constitution. Here, for instance 'one must agree whether health care is a social good that should be distributed fairly by that state' (Bærøe, 2009, p. 55). Then there is (2) the macro level, where 'public health care decisions [are] carried out by government and health care authorities' (2009, p. 55) followed by (3) the meso level, where local priority decisions are taken, and finally (4) the micro level, which is 'the clinical level where consultations between patient and health care workers take place' (Bærøe, 2009, p. 55). Hence, there are a number of factors involved in clinical health care priorities, each of which might influence nursing care for the particular individual. Especially as a consequence of an increasingly sharp tension between distributivist considerations of macro-level allocation and the values that are important at the clinical level of care, lies a danger that the actual values informing professional-care work, such as basic nursing care, might disintegrate. Nurses and health care personnel are increasingly swayed by the imperative to work in a cost-efficient manner, by speeding up 'production' and patient turnover. Therefore, it is ever more important that health care professionals are conscious about their individual responsibility for pursuing the values of their profession.

It is imperative to see in earnest that even minor, day-to-day priority decisions challenge nursing professionals' ethical responsibilities. We should expect an even greater amount of and increasing complexity in these dilemmas in years to come. For instance, the need for nursing care among elderly people will expand rapidly with an increasingly elderly population. At the same time, technological development makes it possible to treat and cure a wide range of diseases.

Besides being a political subject, questions of health care priorities are a growing challenge for the health care professions. Philosophical inquiry can play a role in clarifying the normative value of various distributivist considerations on the different levels of care that Bærøe (2009) emphasises. My focus in this book is theoretical and primarily that of moral philosophy in relation to nurses' daily clinical priority decisions. More precisely, I will base my arguments on different positions and theories that have addressed the issue of partiality and impartiality in ethics.[6] But before I discuss the arguments, let me say a few words about the book's structure.

In Chapter 1 I will present and discuss three levels of impartiality that have significance in nursing care. I will also give an account of the notion of partiality as it is frequently understood in the ethics literature, and then explain how partiality in nursing is to be understood in this book. Chapter 2 is mainly focused on how professional ethics and a comprehension of role-morality account for partiality in nursing care. However, the nursing profession would not exist if it wasn't for patients' needs. Therefore, it seem reasonable to say that, in quite general terms, needs are what guide nursing practice. But patients' needs may be complex, involving both objective and subjective needs, something which can make assessment, decision-making and prioritizing challenging. In Chapter 3 I try to come to terms with some of these complexities, and point towards an analytical and normative implement of importance for the further discussion of partiality. Then, in the fourth and fifth chapter, I explore how partiality in nursing can be justified by two positions advocating a normative value of relationships. In Chapter 4 I discuss a general account of care ethics and the virtue-based arguments for mature care. Then, in Chapter 5, I turn to Samuel Scheffler's (2001; 2010) argument for the normative significance of relationships. I will, however, argue that these accounts fail to address the particularities of professional ethics. The discussion in this fifth chapter ends with a defence of a role-related prerogative for partiality in nursing care. The argument made is that this prerogative is legitimised because of the normative significance that relational proximity has for nursing care. Chapter 6 moves on with a discussion of how this prerogative for partiality can be balanced with justice according to the principle of formal justice. Here, I will argue that decisions from a meso level should not demand that impartiality always trumps partiality. These discussions have implications for the debates about partiality and impartiality in moral philosophy in general. First, while moral philosophy has provided convincing arguments for some forms of partiality within personal relationships and attachments, not much attention has been given to partiality within role contexts and as part of role relationships and obligations. Within the context of professional role relationships I will argue that actions of partiality might be morally desirable, and that the undesirable consequences of partiality should be considered (only) as blameless wrongdoing. In the final chapter I explore how nursing ethics can be adapted for permissible partiality.

Notes

1   This doesn't allude to standardised norms or rules explicating specific criteria for judging what it takes for caring to be adequate. Instead, 'adequate' only entails that nursing care is provided in a way and by means sufficient to satisfy an individual patient's nursing care needs, and this will vary from patient to patient according to his or her (objective and subjective) needs.

2 See for instance Woodward (1999); West et al. (2005); Tadd et al. (2006); Woolhead
   et al. (2006); Nortvedt et al. (2008); Pedersen et al. (2008); Schubert et al. (2008);
   Kalisch et al. (2009); Lucero et al. (2010); Tønnessen et al. (2011), Aiken et al.
   (2012); Zander et al. (2013); Papastravou et al. (2014).
3 See for instance West et al. (2005); Kalisch et al. (2009); Lucero et al. (2010); Aiken
   et al. (2012); Zander et al. (2013); Papastravou et al. (2014)
4 See for instance Nortvedt (1996); Nortvedt et al. (2011); Raustøl (2010); Blum
   (1994).
5 More on this in Chapter 2.
6 I take impartiality here to imply giving equal concern for all patients on the basis of
   their need for health care, as well as maximising nursing care for all who have a
   relevant claim for such care. More on this can be found in Chapter 1.

References

Aiken, L., Sermeus, W., Van den Heede, K., Sloane, D. M., Busse, R., McKee, M.,
  Bruyneel, L., Rafferty, A., Griffiths, P., Tishelman, C., Moreno-Casbas, M.-T., Scott,
  A., Brzostek, T., Schwendimann, R., Schoonhoven, L., Zikos, D., StrømsengS.,
  Ingeborg-Smith, H., and Kutney-Lee, A., 2012. Patient safety, satisfaction, and qual-
  ity of hospital care: Cross sectional surveys of nurses and patients in 12 countries in
  Europe and the United States. *British Medical Journal*, 344, p. e1717.
Annas, J., 1993. *The morality of happiness*. Oxford: Oxford University Press.
Bærøe, K., 2009. Delegated discretion: A call for reasonableness in surrogate decision-
  making and clinical judgment. Dissertation, University of Bergen.
Blum, L., 1994. *Moral perception and particularity*. Cambridge: Cambridge University
  Press.
Holm, S., 2011. Can 'giving preference to my patients' be explained as a role related
  duty in public health care systems? *Health Care Analysis*, 19(1), pp. 89–97.
Kalisch, B., Landstrom, G. and Williams, R., 2009. Missed nursing care: Errors of
  omission. *Nursing Outlook*, 57(1), pp. 3–9.
Lucero, R., Lake, E. and Aiken, L., 2010. Nursing care quality and adverse events in
  US hospitals. *Journal of Clinical Nursing*, 19, pp. 2185–2195.
Nortvedt, P., 1996. *Sensitive judgment: Nursing, moral philosophy and an ethics of care*.
  Oslo: Tano Aschehoug.
Nortvedt, P., Hem, M. and Skirbekk, H., 2011. The ethics of care: Role obligations
  and moderate partiality in health care. *Nursing Ethics*, 18(2), pp. 192–200.
Nortvedt, P., Pedersen, R., Grøthe, K. H., Nordhaug, M., Kirkevold, M., Slettebø,
  Å., Brinchmann, B. S. and Andersen, B., 2008. Clinical prioritisations of healthcare
  for the aged: Professional roles. *Journal of Medical Ethics*, 34(5), pp. 332–335.
Papastavrou, E., Andreou , P. and Vryonides, S., 2014. The hidden ethical element of
  nursing care rationing. *Nursing Ethics*, 21, pp. 583–593.
Pedersen, R., Nortvedt, P., Nordhaug, M., Slettebø, Å., Grøthe, K. H., Kirkevold,
  M., Brinchmann, B. S. and Andersen, B., 2008. In quest of justice? Clinical prior-
  itisation in health care for the aged. *Journal of Medical Ethics*, 34(4), pp. 230–235.
Pettersen, T., 2006. Omsorg som etisk teori. *Norsk Filosofisk Tidsskrift*, no. 2, pp. 151–163
  [Norwegian].
Scheffler, S., 2001. *Boundaries and allegiances*. Oxford: Oxford University Press.
Scheffler, S., 2010. *Equality and tradition*. New York: Oxford University Press.
Schubert, M., Glass, T. R., Clarke, S. P., Aiken, L. H., Schaffert-Witvliet, B., Sloane,
  D. M. and De Geest, S., 2008. Rationing of nursing care and its relationship to

patient outcomes: The Swiss extension of the International Hospital Outcomes Study. *International Journal for Quality in Health Care*, 20(4), pp. 227–237.

Tadd, W., Clarke, A., Lloyd, L., Leino-Kilpi, H., Strandell, C., Lemonidou, C., Petsios, K., Sala, R., Barazzetti, G., Radaelli, S., Zalewski, Z., Bialecka, A., van der Arend, A. and Heymans, R., 2006. The value of nurses' codes: European nurses' views. *Nursing Ethics*, 13(4), pp. 376–393.

The ICN Code of Ethics for Nurses, 2006. www.icn.ch/images/stories/documents/about/icncode_english.pdf [Accessed 14 July 2012].

Tønnessen, S., Nortvedt, P. and Førde, R., 2011. Rationing home-based nursing care: Professional ethical implications. *Nursing Ethics*, 18(3), pp. 386–396.

West, E., Barron, D. and Reeves, R., 2005. Overcoming the barriers to patient-centred care: Times, tools and training. *Journal of Clinical Nursing*, 14(4), pp. 435–443.

Woodward, V., 1999. Achieving moral health care: The challenge of patient partiality. *Nursing Ethics*, 6(5), pp. 390–398.

Woolhead, G., Tadd, W., Boix-Ferrer, J. A., Krajcik, S., Schmid-Pfahler, B., Spjuth, B., Stratton, D., Dieppe, P. and Dignity and Older Europeans (DOE) Project, 2006. 'Tu' or 'Vous?' A European qualitative study of dignity and communication with older people in health and social care settings. *Patients Education and Counseling*, 61(3), pp. 636–671.

World Medical Association, 1948/2006. WMA Declaration of Geneva [Online]. Available at: www.wma.net/en/30publications/10policies/g1/ [Accessed 28 January 2013].

Zander, B., Dobler, L. and Busse, R., 2013. The introduction of DRG funding and hospital nurses' changing perceptions of their practice environment, quality of care and satisfaction: Comparison of cross-sectional surveys over a 10-year period. *International Journal of Nursing Studies*, 50, pp. 219–229.

1 Partiality and impartiality in nursing care

Impartiality and distributive justice in clinical nursing care

As nurses fulfil an institutional role, they are expected to be impartial in distributing nursing care. In this book impartiality is tied to ideas of distributive justice.[1] As said in the introduction, I take impartiality to imply giving equal concern for all patients on the basis of their need for health care, as well as maximising nursing care for all with a relevant need and claim for such care. For the sake of convenience, let us term these notions as 'the rule of equality' and 'the rule of maximising care', respectively.

Imagine a nurse, Kate, who is responsible for the nursing care of five patients in a hospital ward. Kate is expected to distribute nursing care to these five patients impartially. As will be further argued in the second chapter of this book, nurses should, for instance, not distribute care according to gender differences or certain personal preferences or prejudices. This would be considered an example of bias both from the perspective of impartiality, and also from the perspective of partiality, as I will define it. So what does impartiality amount to in nursing care?

Brad Hooker (2010) has identified three levels for directing (moral) impartial assessments: (1) one may assess whether (good) moral rules are applied impartially; (2) one should use impartial benevolence as the single, direct guide to practical decision-making; and (3) from an impartial point of view, one could assess the content of first-order (good) moral rules. This is far from capturing the whole story about impartiality. My purpose here is simply to outline what I take to be the main aspects of impartiality as a component of justice in nursing care.[2]

Impartial application of moral rules

When one is guided solely by the distinctions identified as relevant by a certain rule, one is impartially applying that rule. This is how Hooker (2010) characterises impartial application of first-level moral rules, i.e. the level of practical decision-making. Note that Hooker discusses the impartial *application* of the rule. Hence, the content of the rule does not have to demand impartiality. In this sense, impartiality is considered as a formal component of morality. Applying a rule impartially is not, according to Hooker, incompatible with the compliance with a rule of non-impartial content. Accordingly, impartial application of a rule could include compliance with rules that specify who is benefited or harmed (and to what extent), as well as rules which do not make such distinctions. The rules against lying, stealing, and breaking the law are instantiations of the latter (Hooker, 2010). Impartial compliance with, for instance, the rule against breaking promises implies never breaking a promise to anyone (Hooker, 2010). Hooker then suggests examples of rules which describe who should benefit or be harmed. An instantiation of such a rule is one which states that friends and family should receive a fixed amount when you allocate your own resources (Hooker, 2010).

An important insight here is that partiality can be legitimate at the practical level of impartial assessment. Such a view is also in line with Brian Barry's (1995) idea of first-order impartiality. Barry argues that partiality might be permissible at this level of practical decision-making and action in daily life. According to Barry, a proper distinction between first-order and second-order impartiality is central for the discussion of partiality and impartiality. Indeed, he argues that the debates between partialists and impartialists would be dismissed if this distinction were made properly. Barry argues that on a general level impartiality is and should be required. I return to this in a short while. The problem is that debates on partiality and impartiality most often deal with our private moral lives. Barry points out that those who occupy institutional roles should be committed to a higher degree of impartiality in their decisions and actions. As for the example of the nurse, Kate, it is important to bear in mind that she governs the distribution of public, collective resources, not her own, personal resources. This particular fact is a compelling reason for why those who occupy an institutional role are supposed to be impartial. Hence, even if we accept the claim made by both Hooker and Barry, that partiality might be permissible at the practical level in everyday life, partiality seems to require another sort of justification for professional life.

Let us again consider Hooker's account of impartial application of (first-order) moral rules. Take the rather general rule that 'any nurse should provide adequate and individualised nursing care to those in need of it'. An impartial application of this rule requires that anyone with a need for nursing care should receive (adequate and individualised) nursing care. If Kate sees to it that, say, three out of the five patients receive adequate and individualised nursing care, she does not apply this rule impartially. Imagine then another rule stating that only patients under the age of 90 years should receive nursing care. If two out of Kate's five patients were above this age limit, an impartial application of this rule consists of not attending to the nursing care needs of these two patients. This is so because the rule itself impels Kate to act according to the age limit. That is, the rule itself defines who should benefit. If she nevertheless provides (adequate and individualised) nursing care to all these five patients, she is not applying the rule impartially. Fortunately, this second rule is not very likely to arise in the real world – it is hardly a good moral rule. For the sake of the contention here, we could say that to qualify as a *good* moral rule, the rule has to be impartially defensible (Hooker, 2010). Hooker's argument is that for a rule to be impartially defensible (and thereby good, according to Hooker), it must give equal weight to the good of all parties involved. This leads us to Hooker's second approach to comprehending impartiality.

Impartial benevolence and practical reasoning

Hooker argues for impartial benevolence as the only direct determiner of everyday practical decision-making. This is an (act-)utilitarian approach for making impartial assessments. In this sense impartial benevolence should be understood as equal concern for the good of each (Hooker, 2010). Equal concern for the good of each, Hooker argues, implies that benefit or harm to one individual have the same-size benefit or harm to any other individual. According to Hooker this form of impartial assessment is only sometimes appropriate in our ordinary everyday lives. In fact, if the notion of impartial benevolence was interpreted literally, the results might be somewhat absurd, as Hooker writes:

> You might know more about how to benefit your family and friends than you know how to benefit strangers. Thus you might attend to your family and friends more than to others – but not because you have greater concern for your family and friends. On the contrary, whenever you were sure that doing something for a stranger would benefit the stranger at least a little more than doing the same thing for yourself or your family member or friend, you would benefit the stranger. If you could save three lives by giving to one person one of your kidneys, to the second person the other of your kidneys, and to the third person your heart, you would do so.
>
> (Hooker, 2010, p. 31)

But impartial benevolence is required, he argues, if one is occupying certain official roles. However, is it not the case that a requirement to maximise net aggregate benefit would be too demanding in certain official roles, such as in nursing care? Hooker acknowledges that unconstrained impartiality could sometimes be inappropriate even in official roles. For instance, there are deontological prohibitions against murder, torture, robbery, and fraud (Hooker, 2010). To point out extreme actions such as torture and robbery as exceptions to the utilitarian claim is not very helpful for my purpose here. The choice between, say, fraud and impartial benevolence, is not likely to arise in the context of nursing care. It is more likely that, for instance, a deontological restriction against harming might *conflict* with impartial benevolence. In health care, a principle of not harming is fundamental. Simultaneously, some form and some degree of harm is unavoidable. For instance, as

Edwards (1996) points out, a surgeon inflicts physical harm on a patient undergoing an appendectomy when he cuts open the patient's abdomen. One can also imagine the harm inflicted on a mentally ill patient who is (legally) forced into medical treatment or hospital admission (Edwards, 1996). In such cases, a prohibition against harming the patients as an avoidable part of the procedure is (at least ordinarily) ruled out by concern for the good of the patients. In other words, harming a patient may in certain situations be the precondition for benefiting the patient.

In other situations, there is an absolute prohibition against harming patients. The problem is that it is not always obvious how to comprehend the notion of harm. Consider Kate again. Let us say that one of her patients suffers from unstable diabetes mellitus and needs an injection of insulin one hour prior to breakfast. Suppose also that this patient is demented, though competent enough to give consent, and moreover refuses the injection. As a result, Kate may need quite lot of time to deal with this situation. She must communicate efficiently with this patient, assess the patient's blood sugar, discuss the situation with the physician, and so on. If Kate could maximise net aggregate benefit for her five patients by postponing the injection of insulin, is she morally permitted (or even required) to do so? Not so if the patient is physically harmed[3] by not getting the injection. This is due to the severity of need. If the severity of this patient's need overrides the other patients' (net aggregate) needs, a prohibition against postponing this situation rules out impartial benevolence.

Imagine then another nurse, Jason. As a community nurse on nightshift, Jason is responsible for the nursing care needs of fifteen patients. If Jason could maximise the net benefit of all these patients by putting sanitary pads onto three of the patients (in order to save the time it would have taken to take these patients to the bathroom), should he do so? There is no deontological prohibition against the action itself. But there is a prohibition against harming patients. The question is whether Jason harms these three patients if he chooses to do so. Suppose none of these patients would refuse to wear sanitary pads, say, because they are severely demented and have lost the ability to cognitively grasp their situations. In a radical sense, then, one might say that these patients would not suffer if they were to use pads instead of going to the toilet. Their needs are not ignored, one may say. In that sense, Jason is not breaking the deontological prohibition against harming since the rule does not seem to apply to the situation. If this is so, he should act according to the principle of impartial benevolence. But I would object to this conclusion. After all, is not humiliation and disrespect for patients' integrity as harmful as the physical harm that might be caused by having a wet pad the whole night through? Indeed, this is the core of the ethical problem facing Jason: On what grounds should someone's right to adequate and individualised nursing care be violated more than someone else's? The point here is that harm can take many forms. Any assessment of harm also requires contextual sensitivity. Therefore, it might turn out that a deontological prohibition against harming frequently conflicts with or even rules out impartial benevolence. But this does not in itself imply that the rule of impartial benevolence falls short of being a good moral rule. It only shows that impartial benevolence is challenged as a prima facie rule. In the third section of Chapter 5 I return to the challenging claims of consequentialism (and utilitarianism) and the possible deontological restrictions against it.

Impartial assessment of moral rules and action

At the level of practical decision-making we saw that impartiality leaves some scope for partial action. More precisely, one is permitted to follow partial rules as long as these rules are applied impartially. Hooker's worry seems to be that one ends up favouring rules that are partial. Therefore, he argues that the rule upon which one acts should be impartially justified (Hooker, 2010). He asserts that good moral rules are those that place equal value on the good of all people involved.

There are of course other approaches for impartial assessments than that of Hooker's rule consequentialism. One is the view that impartial justification is ensured if the principle (upon which one acts) cannot be reasonably rejected by any individual.[4] This is Barry's contractarian view of second-order impartiality. As referred to above, Barry argues that partiality is permissible at the level of practical decision-making and action. But at the level of principles, one should ensure impartial justification. This is also the level at which the degree of partiality should be refined (Barry, 1995). According to this idea, institutions should be arranged in a way that anyone reasonably would accept. In health care, impartiality is directed both to health care receivers and to health care providers. For instance, the superior and macro level of health care should ensure that every citizen acquires certain basic rights to health care. At the same time, certain principles and rules are developed at this level as to ensure health care professionals act according to patients' rights.[5] According to Barry's position, then, we must reasonably expect that anyone would accept either kind of principle.

Consider again the rule[6] where 'only patients under the age of 90 years old should receive nursing care'. Previously I said that this rule is not a good moral rule. Why is this so? For one thing, it is intuitively absurd. Besides, according to Barry's account of second-order impartiality, it is not likely that anyone would reasonably accept it.[7] Second, it contravenes what I called the 'rule of equality' (i.e. equal concern for all patients on the basis of their need for health care). Let us for a moment call these two rules R^1 and R^2, respectively. According to Hooker's position, R^1 would not qualify as a good moral rule since it does not apply equal concern to the good of each person involved. Why then, is R^2 a good moral rule? According to Hooker's account, it surely is. That is, for an impartial justification we should ask the questions: 'impartial with respect to what and with regard to whom?' As for R^2 the answer is 'impartial with regard to needs of health care and with regard to any patient'. R^2 then states that each patient should be accorded equal concern for his or her health care needs (implying equal respect for all patients' needs). This rather general rule seems to correspond with Hooker's account of a good moral rule. Could R^2 be impartially justified at the level of principles (i.e. as second-order impartiality)? Most probably yes. The basic premise for impartial justification is that no one would reasonably reject the principle. Health care is a collective good from which everyone benefits, more or less, during their lifetime. The principle should therefore hold equally for everyone. Health care institutions that adapt R^2 therefore seem to meet the demands of second-order impartiality.

Nevertheless, a higher-level impartial justification does not guarantee an impartial *application* of the principle, nor does it require it. As Raustøl points out:

> Even though I give some special weight to the good of my friend in my practical deliberation, I am only justified in doing so if I can defend the rule upon which I am acting against the requirement that this rule, if widely accepted, would tend to give equal importance to the good of each. In this way, argues the indirect impartialist, the agent can care about the other for his own sake, and still respect impartiality.
>
> (Raustøl, 2010, p. 35)

Another way of putting this is to say that if I (as a nurse) think I am right in giving special attention to one of the patients I am responsible for, I must accept that any other nurse also is right in giving special attention to one of her patients. But note that this right, if accepted, is a right of nurses, not of patients. In that case we should say that if I (as a patient) think I have the right to special attention, then I must accept that any other patient also has this right. Theoretically, such rights can be impartially justified both from Hooker's account and from Barry's account. The problem is how to deal with the practical implications, especially situations of scarce resources. This is not a problem exclusively for impartialists, though.

As we have seen, moral impartiality can be comprehended on three levels. The rest of this chapter consists of an analysis of the notion of partiality.

The notion of partiality

Partial acts and partial standings

In the ethics literature, partiality is generally understood as special attentiveness, responsiveness, and favouritism between or among those who are considered to be close (Friedman, 1991, p. 818).[8] Scheffler, for instance, argues that partiality is '[a] preferential stand or fondness or affection for a particular person or group of persons' (Scheffler, 2010, p. 42). The debates on partiality and impartiality in ethics seem to treat the motivational ground for partiality and actions of partiality alike. That is, usually, what explains partial standing towards a person is also what explains a corresponding partial act to the benefit of this person. This represents the most common way to comprehend partiality in ethics. Arguments for partiality are traditionally established on the idea that personal relationships with people we love or care about have an intrinsic normative value that in itself provides us with reasons for partiality. Scheffler is a prominent proponent of partiality based on valuable relationships. One of his main arguments is that valuing a personal relationship in itself gives reasons for partiality: 'Interpersonal relationships could not play the role they do in our lives, and in some cases could not even exist, unless they were treated by the participants as providing such reasons' (Scheffler, 2001, p. 121). According to such a view, partiality is a means for protecting something of moral value, such as our personal relationships. If a partial standing based on valuable relationships represents a normative source,[9] we must ask whether this source is morally legitimate as a reason for partial acts in professional ethics. Even though it might be so in our ordinary lives, it is doubtful whether this is so in professional contexts such as nursing care. Moreover, there is an important difference between explaining and justifying reasons for action. Although, for instance, as we shall see, Scheffler (2001; 2010) has provided normative arguments justifying partiality this way, partiality in professional contexts like nursing needs another kind of justification.

The question then is, of course, based on the reasons in which partiality can be justified in professional care. This implies asking what partiality aims to protect in nursing care. I return to this later in the chapter, and it is also a central point for discussion in Chapter 5. Crucial to my claim is that partiality in the professional context of nursing should concern partiality towards patients' nursing care needs, not towards particular patients as private persons. This is not to say that nurses should consider patients as objects with needs that can be separated from the sick and needy human being in his or her totality. It should only be taken to imply that it is the patient's objective and subjective nursing care needs, not the patient as a private person, that are central to the question of partiality in nursing care. This also means that where partiality in our ordinary lives concerns both persons qua private persons and our relationships with them, and/or their interests and needs, only the latter, and with regard to nursing care needs, is relevant for my argument. This point is magnified if we are to avoid arbitrary partiality based on prejudice and personal preferences such as liking or disliking someone. More on this will be discussed in a short while.

I aim to establish an argument for partiality that is not premised on a valuable (personal) relationship between nurse and patient. In other words, I will argue that partiality is not necessarily presupposed by a *pre-existing partial standing* towards the person to whom one acts partially. And vice versa: a partial standing towards a person does not necessarily lead to partial behaviour. This means that one can act partially towards someone without having a pre-existing partial standing towards that person. It also means that one can have a partial standing towards a person without thereby acting partially towards that person. Although these are claims that mainly call for empirical investigation, the analytical distinction between acts and motivation is in itself important when discussing the normative legitimacy of partiality in professional contexts.

Let me further illustrate my point concerning the relation, or rather the distinction, between partial acts and partial standing by the use of a classic example commonly referred to in debates on partiality and impartiality. The example is formulated by Peter Singer:

> if I am walking past a shallow pond and see a child drowning in it, I ought to wade in and pull the child out. This will mean getting my clothes muddy, but this is insignificant, while the death of the child would presumably be a very bad thing.
>
> (Singer, 1972, p. 231)

Singer uses this example in contrast to our hesitation to donate only a small amount of money to save the life of one or many refugees far off. His example emphasises an important aspect of partiality, namely our inclination to favour those who are *physically close to us in time and space*. In this example, however, there is no assumption, nor any presupposition, that we need to have a pre-existing partial *standing* based on a personal relationship towards those of whom we are partial. Besides, being partial towards a particular person's needs and interests does not necessarily entail being partial to that person in general (as a partial standing based on a relationship to that person).

In order to justify this point further, we could articulate two different categories of partial standings.[10] One is a partial standing based on close personal relationships. In that case there is a partial standing towards the person in his or her totality, as is typically the case in parental partiality and friendship. Partial standing based on close personal relationships seems to endure distances like physical or geographical space. Suppose, for instance, that my sister works in Afghanistan for Doctors Without Borders. Since I know the winters can be very cold in the area of Afghanistan where she lives, I buy her a warm winter coat for Christmas. This costs me a total sum of 2,000 NOK. I also donate 200 NOK to Doctors Without Borders. This could easily qualify as a partial act since I spend a far greater sum on my sister, who presumably could have bought her own warm winter clothes, than I do on charitable work for poor people who cannot afford clothes that keep them warm. This partial act is based on my close personal relationship with my sister. And it endures the distance between us.

The other form of partial standing is based on a sense of belonging to a group, society, neighbourhood, nation, etc.[11] This partial standing is not directed towards particular and identified persons, but to any other person considered part of our group. In these cases there need not be any *close personal* relationship from which partiality arises. In so far as the person saving the drowning child acts out of a partial standing, it is a partial standing based on a sense of belonging to the same neighbourhood or society. But it seems more likely that the person acts as he does because of the immediacy of the situation, not because of any pre-existing partial standing towards the child. He witnesses something terrible and is able to help. There is something valuable at stake, *here* and *now*.

But why does it then qualify as a partial act? In other words, if we reject a pre-existing partial standing towards the one who benefits as a necessary element in partiality, what then characterises partiality? Let me try to illuminate my point by using another example. Suppose I have to choose between either doing (a) or doing (b). Also suppose that (a) and (b) are equally desirable and valuable from some objective point of view. Doing (a) would benefit my best friend, and doing (b) would benefit some unknown other. If I choose to do (a), am I then acting partially towards my best friend? That depends, one may say, on what reasons I have for choosing (a) instead of (b). If one holds the view that partial acts are done out of partial standings (here, based on a valuable relationship), my partial standing towards my friend seems to be the explanation for doing (a). But what if I choose (b) instead of (a) – am I then acting partially towards the unknown other? Or does the absence of a partial standing towards this unknown other disqualify (b) as a partial act? One can act partially without being motivated by a pre-existing partial standing towards the one who benefits. Suppose my choice in a particular situation is shaped by equal concern for the good of each, not by favour. If we hold the view that this is what motivates and causes my choice of action, then some-one could say that my choice is *not* partial, but rather an impartial choice resulting in (fair) differential treatment. Since both (a) and (b) are equally desirable and valuable from some objective point of view, we cannot expect any objective, discernible differences between them. Choices (a) and (b) may require different courses of action, but still may be equally desirable and valuable. I make a choice based on some calculation of equal concern for the good of my friend and the good of the unknown other. In this case, I am not acting partially.

But let us instead say I choose (a) because I have the ability here and now to do (a), and doing (b) seems to require that I change my plans for the next hour. Quite often, I think, we make decisions based on practical reasoning like this. Besides, I am not (necessarily) doing something morally bad or wrong by acting from such a reason. But neither have I established a reason for why this choice is (morally) right. The case in point here is that this choice can result in acts we conceive as arbitrary or unfair. If I chose to do (a) instead of (b) for no other reason than convenience for myself, I am not acting *impartially*. Rather, it is an illustration of partiality towards one's own inter-ests, but not based on a pre-existing partial standing towards the person who benefits from my choice.

Although partiality does not need to be arbitrary and unfair (as I will argue later), this is an intuitive way of characterising choices like this. This is perhaps one of the most important distinctions between partiality and impartial differential treatment. My main point here is that partiality appears arbitrary and/or unfair because, from an agent-neutral point of view, there are no qualitative (or quantitative) differences between the options presented. Saving the drowning child, but, say, refusing to donate money that could save the life of a child far off, is a partial act – not because it is characterised by a partial standing, but because the lives of two children are of equal value. Hence, the choice of action appears (and also is) unfair, perhaps also arbitrary. The challenge to accept, then, is how to establish an argument for legitimate partiality that is not premised on unfairness or arbitrariness (even though it might appear to be so). Later I aim to establish such an argument.

Now, although it might be true that we have an inclination to favour those who are close to us in time and space (as is Singer's point), this is usually expressed as being partial to these persons' needs and interests in certain situations. It is usually not the case that we are partial to them in general (as is the case in personal relationships), which would mean a partial standing towards all their interests and needs. Saving the child from drowning is not premised on any form of relationship to this child; the child might be a total stranger towards whom you have no general partial standing. It is not the case, for instance, that you favour this child's need and interests of other kinds and in other situations. Perhaps you, say, prefer to spend your spare time on local charitable work instead of taking this child to her handball practice even though you know this would have meant a lot to that child. As Singer points out, we hesitate when we are asked to donate some money to save the life of a faraway child who is as equally unknown to us as the drowning child. This noticeable and peculiar discrepancy is also Singer's point when he questions the normative significance of physical closeness to the needy. Being physically near to a person, as in having personal contact with that person, may, Singer argues, make it more likely that we shall assist that person. But according to Singer, physical closeness does not in it self legitimise that we ought to help the person physically near to us rather than a person who happens to be far away.

I have said that a partial standing does not necessarily lead to partial acts. To be more precise, we could say that a partial standing *should* not always lead to partial acts. Having a pre-existing partial standing does not necessarily make it morally legitimate to act on this predisposition. Suppose I have a general partial standing towards my best friend because of our valuable relationship. The partial standing I have towards my best friend does not always make it morally legitimate for me to be partial towards his needs and interests. Sometimes my best friend's needs and interests collide or conflict with those of other people. If other people's needs in a situation are more severe than my friend's needs at a particular moment, I might not be permitted to be partial to my friend's needs, despite my partial standing. Besides, in some cases the reasons we are partial are not always evident (for instance, is it for the sake of the friend or the friendship, or for the sake of the particular need, or for both, or none of these?). Nevertheless, the link between partial standing and partial acts perhaps provides a strong case for partialists: Partiality is deeply human and natural, and it protects those things of moral value to us. But at the same time it is perhaps exactly this perspective that lends credence to an argument against partiality: Partiality is unfair with regard to those who are not in privileged positions to benefit from partiality. And it is also, as we shall see in a while, the main reason for why relationship-based arguments for partiality in professional ethics are problematic.

Partiality in professional care does not presuppose a *pre-existing partial standing* in any of the forms mentioned above, and one must distinguish between partiality as an act and partiality as a special standing or fondness. Most important here, when asserting the normative significance of proximity as action-guiding in professional contexts, it is imperative to take into account impartial concerns of distributive justice. But that said, my point at this moment is that being partial can mean acting on reasons other than a pre-existing partial standing towards the person (qua person) who benefits from the partial act.

This reasoning is in line with Reader's (2003) account of partiality based on real encounters. Reader argues that partialists are right in thinking that (only) relational properties ground moral obligations, but wrong in the *kinds* of relational properties they have hitherto singled out. To be morally obligating, Reader says, other partialists believe that a relationship must be 'socially recognised' or 'valued' by the parties. But to Reader, the important point here is that a relationship is a real connection between an agent and something else, and she criticises partialists for relying more on shared properties than what is actually between them. Moral obligations then, according to Reader, are powerful even in rudimentary relationships like encounters: 'When needing others loom large here and now, they place considerable moral obligations on an agent' (Reader, 2003, p. 377).

Reader's account of relationships bears some resemblance to care ethics, as well as to Scheffler's account of the notion of relationships, which will be topics for discussion in Chapter 5. The similarity between the two is the emphasis on the moral obligation and responsibility that arises from relationships. To Reader, it is what she calls 'the real connection' that obligates agents. This real connection can take many forms, one of which is presence: '[W]e recognise that when someone collapses in front of me, I am obligated to help [her] be the real connection between us that is our presence to each other' (Reader, 2003, p. 372). Other such forms are biology, history, environment, practice, projects (Reader, 2003). All these forms have in common the feature of holding the related together and constituting the relationship.

In brief, then, Reader's account of partiality from encounter is a broader concept than partiality from personal bonds and attachments. We could say that Reader's account of a real connection is not dependent on any pre-existing shared properties. Instead, it could be a here-and-now situation, where one person is confronted with another being's immediate need for assistance. It is within this encounter that one has the ability to help the other in some way or another. And it is from this real connection that moral obligation arises. This does not mean that one cannot and should not respond to the needs of others. The important point here is that this real connection, this confrontation with another's need, is not dependent on the non-instrumental value of the connection or the relationship between the parties involved. According to Reader, moral obligation can arise from any such encounter (and not just certain valuable personal relationships) as long as there is a real connection between the parties.

It is also worth mentioning that partiality can imply favouring someone or something in such a way that others are ignored or excluded. Their interests may be ignored, and their needs may not be met (adequately). But in a more moderate version, partiality implies giving priority to someone or something over someone or something else. In this sense, those who are not prioritised are not totally ignored or excluded. I will not argue for a version of partiality that *ignores* patients' needs for nursing care to the benefit of only a few patients. My aim is to argue for a version of partiality that aspires to ensure adequate and individualised nursing care. This may have some unavoidable and undesirable consequences for other patients, but never to the extent that their needs for nursing care are totally ignored.

When I worked on this topic, I realised that the notion of partiality within the context of nursing was a controversial topic. At best the combination appeared counterintuitive to many people; at worst it appeared immoral. Hence, in discussing my research with people, I often felt compelled to explain my particular conception of partiality – or even more importantly, the way I do *not* conceive of partiality in nursing care. Partiality can be understood in at least two different ways. For one, partiality can imply prejudice or bias, which is always incompatible with morality. But partiality can also imply a special responsibility that sometimes (or always) is either morally permissible or morally required. Initially, it is this latter form of partiality that I focus on in this book. However, in both instances, partiality means particular concern for certain people and/or for the interests and needs of certain people over other people and/or their interests and needs. Though disfavouring is usually not considered as partiality, we should pay attention to this way of conceiving of partiality in both the forms mentioned here. The decisive element that distinguishes these two forms of partiality – i.e. prejudice or bias versus social responsibility – concerns the *reasons* for partiality. The next two subsections aim to describe two different conceptions of partiality, and to clarify how partiality is conceived of in this book. As will be shown, I will argue for professional partiality that is conceived differently than the more personal partiality referenced in most debates about partiality. This implies that reasons of partiality in both forms mentioned are somewhat different in professional contexts.

Partiality and prejudice

Intuitively, I think, most people associate partiality with something undesirable and illegitimate, as something unfair. In this sense, acting partially means acting on prejudice and favouring someone unfairly. Social, racial, and religious prejudices are good examples of the kind of partiality that is particularly damaging and immoral.

Holm delineates three ways discrimination can connote favouring a certain person. This is a useful way to distinguish between different forms of partiality. First, if discrimination means giving unjust preference, it follows, Holm says, that health care professionals should not discriminate. But this guideline does not really tell us much, since, as Holm emphasises, though it is an analytical truth, it still leaves open the question of 'locating the unjustifiable injustice' (2011, p. 90).

This first connotation also shows that defining 'partiality' with the connation of discrimination in health care is a misconstruction. Second, discrimination may connote 'giving preference to'. A central question then is, according to Holm, whether it is true that health care professionals never should discriminate. For instance, Bærøe and Bringedal (2011) argue for increased attention to socioeconomic factors (SEF) and the socioeconomic status (SES) of patients. They argue that equitable health care must give consideration to the impact of socioeconomic factors:

> Remaining neutral towards patients' SES in this respect does not promote equal regard. It follows that priority setting on the basis of socio-economic factors is required in fair clinical distribution of care, e.g. through allocating more time to patients with low SES (61 ord).
>
> (Bærøe and Bringedal, 2011, p. 526)

Their argument is that socioeconomic, non-medical concerns are relevant as a ground for partiality, or 'giving preference to'. These are relevant concerns because socioeconomic factors imply differences in how patients gain benefit from treatment. This is, therefore, an important argument for how partiality might be justifiable, based on non-medical criteria.

The third connotation of discrimination Holm refers to is showing 'preference against'. Holm writes:

> But this does not settle the matter against giving preference to some patients, because it is not obvious that a health care professional who gives preference to her own patients thereby necessarily shows a preference against those patients that are not hers.
>
> (Holm, 2011, p. 91)

This argument illustrates the importance of the distinction I have referred to between partial standings and partial acts. In health care, partiality can be justified in the context of partial acts, not partial standings. Here it becomes evident that such prejudices also imply *disfavouring* someone directly or indirectly. For example, a female nurse favouring female patients at the expense of male patients, everything all else being equal, displays partiality based on gender discrimination. And if, for instance, a nurse favours taking care of a patient who happens to be a close friend or family member at the expense of another patient, and these two patients' needs are equal, then the nurse is partial in a discriminatory way. Friendship is the quintessential example of partiality, as are other familiar relationships. But the nurse–patient relationship is an institutionalised role relationship where any pre-existing partial standing based on personal relationships should not count as acceptable reasons for partiality. I return to this point soon.

By contrast, a nurse who does not pay adequate attention to the needs of a patient because she does not like the patient personally is also partial in this sense. However, disfavouring someone is not commonly understood as partiality. Still, disfavouring is closely related to illegitimate forms of partiality since it entails neglecting someone's legitimate needs for morally illegitimate reasons. Besides, disfavouring also entails benefiting or favouring *someone else* for immoral reasons. That is, the beneficiaries are favoured, though indirectly, not because of some special concern for them, but because someone else in particular is disfavoured. In professional care, such disfavouring is just as immoral as favouring when the unequal treatment is grounded in prejudices based on a patient's gender, social background, age, etc.

Liking or disliking someone is another illegitimate reason for partiality, or so is my claim. But whereas disliking someone obviously counts as prejudice and bias in nursing care, there are other issues that arise when a nurse takes a particular liking to a patient. Raustøl (2010) argues that as long as a nurse's role-based duties towards all her patients have been discharged, the nurse is permitted to act partially when she likes a certain patient. Raustøl's view implies that a nurse is required to care for any patient, regardless of whether she likes the patient or not. But if the nurse grows to like a patient, she is permitted to be partial to this patient. I am concerned with this claim.[12] It is quite possible that some patients in general are more sympathetic, or in some way easier to like, than other patients. Imagine a patient, Pat, who suffers from cancer, and all the nurses at the hospital ward like her very much. Pat is a sympathetic woman, never requiring much, and is easy to like. Every day, during every shift, all other patients at the ward receive their care. But Pat is always given some extra care because the nurses like her. If resources are scarce, this will probably imply that the other patients only got a minimum of care, whereas Pat might receive a little more, even if someone else (who may be less favoured than Pat, or not liked at all) could benefit more from it. But such implications are probably not what Raustøl would argue for. Raustøl's point seems to me to be that there ought to be some moral space for emotions such as liking and affection, if desirable, to develop in nurse–patient relationships. Perhaps supererogation is what Raustøl alludes to. In this sense, some extra care, or being partial, based on affection and liking, could qualify as actions 'beyond the call of duty' (Dancy, 1993).[13] I will still argue that whether or not the nurse likes the patient, or has any other personal preferences or bonds, should be irrelevant to the care offered.

The case of personal bonds and preferences is somewhat similar to that of liking. Suppose I work in a nursing home ward and one day my grandfather is admitted to this ward. Does my relationship with my grandfather legitimise my partiality towards him and his needs? Had my duties towards the other patients been discharged, it might perhaps be so. But if these duties are not adequately discharged, I am not permitted to be partial to him simply because he is my grandfather. Hence, partiality based on personal relationships like these should, theoretically speaking, only be allowable in a situation where there are enough resources to fulfil the needs of all patients equally.

Consider another example. On my way back from work one day a car accident happens right in front of me. Two patients are quite badly injured and in need of ambulances. One of these patients happens to be my best friend and, after doing the best I can for both of them, I spend the time waiting for the ambulances at my friend's side. When the first ambulance arrives I desperately beg the attending paramedics to prioritise my friend. But suppose, then, that I was not on my way home from work, but instead at work in an emergency ward. Two patients from a car accident arrived, with equal needs for medical treatment and nursing care. One of these patients is my best friend. Am I now to prioritise caring for my best friend, begging the attending physician to give my friend preference? Probably, and hopefully, no one would blame me for being emotionally affected by the situation. But as a nurse on duty, my obligations must be focused on the patients' needs, rather than them as private persons. Later, I will discuss further what could count as a morally relevant reason for unequal treatment (partiality). But it suffices here to say that any prejudice or bias, such as liking or disliking a patient, should not count as a legitimate reason for partiality. Let me now turn to what I conceive of as legitimate forms of partiality.

Partiality and valuable relationships

Typical examples of partiality include parental partiality, such as a mother's favouritism towards her child's needs over the needs of others, and partiality due to friendship. Partiality in this sense usually serves some further moral value: It contributes to sustaining our close relationships or something valuable to us. According to Scheffler (2010), this form of partiality is central to any sensible understanding of morality and moral life.

> at the most fundamental level, the moral reasons that apply to intimates are no different from those that apply to strangers. But once we accept that reasons of partiality are genuine reasons that flow from some of our most basic values and in fact apply to our treatment of intimates, the insistence that these reasons have no direct moral relevance risks making morality itself seem irrelevant.
>
> (Scheffler, 2010, p. 74)

However, as already indicated, in professional contexts, this otherwise morally legitimate form of partiality is much more problematic.

In terms of nursing care it is important to emphasise the moral basis of the argument for impartiality. The patients' needs for nursing care are the motivational[14] and ethical basis for the professional encounter between a nurse and a patient. In other words, without the needs for nursing or medical care, there would be no professional encounter (Nordhaug and Nortvedt, 2011). And these needs should take precedence over any personal preferences of the nurse or the patient. For instance, as I argued above, whether or not the nurse and the patient know each other personally, or happen to like each other, is, and should be, irrelevant to the establishment of the professional encounter between them. Any such preferences should also be irrelevant to the quality of the care provided.[15] But notably, this impartiality is not inconsistent with other forms of more moderate partiality.[16] It is partiality in this particular sense I am interested in here. Since partiality means special and stronger concern for certain people and/or for the interests and needs of certain people than for other people and/or their interests and needs, we must ask which reasons justify partiality in nursing care. In Chapters 4 and 5, I examine different approaches to justifying partiality, and propose an answer to this question.

I will build on the following description of partiality in nursing care: *Partiality means that one patient is given precedence over other patient(s) because of relational proximity between the nurse and this patient.*

It is important to bear in mind that I am discussing partiality within a context of prioritisation. In this sense, the term partiality means the same thing as 'give preference to' and 'give priority to'. Partiality in nursing care might be legitimate if and only if the needs of the patients in question are equal in a morally relevant sense, and I return to this designation in Chapter 6. For example, partiality could imply that it is permissible, and even morally desirable, for a nurse to spend her time at a patient's deathbed even if she could have instead spent the same amount of time, say, by performing the morning toileting of two other patients.

My main argument will be that, in some situations, nurses will not be able to fulfil commitments to providing adequate and individualised nursing care if they are not permitted to be partial. This argument is in some sense in line with Holm's argument that the best way to achieve fairness, impartiality, and justice in health care probably is to permit health care professionals to be partial. But I will also argue that partiality could be permissible even if it in fact does conflict with such values. Throughout this book, nursing care will for the most part be referred to as 'the nursing project'. I return to this topic in Chapters 2 and 5.

Notes

1 This is not to say that justice always and solely depends on impartiality. And as will be shown in this section, impartiality does not necessarily exclude partiality.

2 There are other ways of analysing the moral concept of impartiality in nursing care. For a more thorough analysis of impartiality and nursing care, see for instance Raustøl (2010).

3 More than physical harm is at stake here. The situation also requires assessments of whether the principle of respect for patient's autonomy is ruled out by the duty to provide necessary medical treatment. If so, there is also a question of inflicting harm when forcing the injection on the patient.

4 We might also say that impartiality is ensured if the assessment is carried out from an agent-neutral point of view. Agent-neutral assessment would imply that rules are picked out without any reference to (personal) interests of the agent. Agent-neutrality, or objectivity, is sometimes used interchangeably with impartiality, but refers only to one component of impartiality. More on agent-neutrality is presented in the next chapter.

5 Additionally, professional ethical guidelines and codes, such as the ICN codes, are developed internally in each health care profession.

6 We could also call it the 'principle of equality'. See for instance Edwards (1996) for a four-level, principle-based approach to nursing ethics. According to Edwards, level one refers to particular judgments as instances of moral rules, and level two is the level of the rules of veracity, privacy, confidentiality, and fidelity. Third is the level of the four principles of autonomy – beneficence, nonmaleficence, and justice. The fourth level is the level of ethical theories.

7 While there might be arguments for setting age limits as regards expensive medical treatment and/or life-prolonging medical treatment, these arguments are not applicable to nursing care. For instance, some might argue that over the age of 90 one shouldn't be offered an expensive life-prolonging treatment in the case of a severe illness with a bad prognosis. Instead, they would argue, these patients should be offered adequate nursing care and palliative medical treatment. I cannot imagine any – moral or professional – argument for setting age limits to nursing care. As said above, the idea is absurd.

8 I believe any form of partiality also includes partiality towards non-human animals, groups, communities, nations, personal interests and projects, etc. But since my discussion is restricted to nursing care (and nursing care is directed towards human beings), it suffices here to say that partiality is directed to humans.

9 By normative source I here mean an action-guiding reason. We should, however, bear in mind the distinction between what we believe to be normative sources and what really are normative sources. This distinction relates to what Torbjörn Tännsjö terms the 'Humean notion of practical reasons' and the 'moral notion of practical reasons' (Tännsjö, 2010, p. 3). On the former notion, 'practical reasons are beliefs and desires a person has when acting, which could cause the action' (ibid., p.11), and refers thereby to an explanation of the action. On the moral or normative notion, on the other hand, practical reasons are different in that they explain our obligations: 'I have a moral reason *to* perform a certain action only if I *ought* to perform it. The moral reasons are the facts, if such facts exist, that explain *why* I ought to perform it' (ibid., p. 3). Such a distinction is central for partiality in professional care, where our ordinary intuitions as well as our considered judgments of what counts as legitimate reasons for partiality in our daily lives are not directly transferable to our professional lives.

10 Most often, partiality refers to acts and attitudes at an individual level – i.e. acts or attitudes of individual agents towards individual others. An agent can be partial towards a certain person or a certain group of persons. From this background, reasons for partiality are commonly referred to as agent-relative reasons. But partiality can also refer to acts and attitudes at a collective level in a society, e.g. at a political level or at a collective professional level. We can also find partiality at a global level, for instance a nation's inclination to favour cooperation with certain

other nations, etc. In any of these latter cases, it does not make sense to speak about agent-relative reasons for partiality.

11 See for instance Scheffler (2010) on relationship-dependent reasons and membership-dependent reasons.

12 It is important to bear in mind that questions of partiality are relevant due to resource constraints of some sort.

13 More on supererogation and partiality is presented in Chapter 2.

14 Note that the word 'motivational' here only refers to a normative ideal. To examine what *in fact* motivates nurses in specific situations is a question far beyond the scope of this book.

15 It is of course an empirical question whether or not it is true that personal preferences, economical concerns, etc., influence the treatment or care provided, and the relationship between professionals and patients.

16 As opposed to strict partiality, moderate forms of partiality provide some scope for impartiality.

References

Barry, B., 1995. *A treatise on social justice. Volume II: Justice as impartiality.* Oxford: Clarendon Press.

Bærøe, K. and Bringedal, B., 2011. Just health: On the conditions of acceptable and unacceptable priority settings with respect to patients' socioeconomic status. *Journal of Medical Ethics*, 37(9), pp. 526–529.

Dancy, J., 1993. *Moral reasons.* Oxford: Blackwell.

Edwards, S., 1996. *Nursing ethics: A principled-based approach.* London: Macmillan.

Friedman, M., 1991. The practice of partiality. *Ethics*, 101(4), pp. 818–835.

Holm, S., 2011. Can 'giving preference to my patients' be explained as a role related duty in public health care systems? *Health Care Analysis*, 19(1), pp. 89–97.

Hooker, B., 2010. When is impartiality morally appropriate? In: Feltham, B. and Cottingham, J., eds, *Partiality and impartiality: Morality, special relationships, and the wider world.* New York: Oxford University Press, pp. 26–41.

Nordhaug, M. and Nortvedt, P., 2011. Justice and proximity: Problems for an ethics of care. *Health Care Analysis*, 19, pp. 3–14.

Raustøl, A., 2010. Impartiality and partiality in nursing ethics. s. 1. Dissertation, University of Reading.

Reader, S., 2003. Distance, relationship, and moral obligation. *The Monist*, 86(3), pp. 367–381.

Scheffler, S., 2001. *Boundaries and allegiances.* Oxford: Oxford University Press.

Scheffler, S., 2010. *Equality and tradition.* New York: Oxford University Press.

Singer, P., 1972. Famine, affluence, and morality. *Philosophy and Public Affairs*, 1(1), pp. 229–243.

Stroud, S., 2010. Permissible partiality, projects, and plural agency. In: Feltham, B. and Cottingham, J., eds, *Partiality and impartiality: Morality, special relationships, and the wider world.* Oxford: Oxford University Press, pp. 131–150.

Tännsjö, T., 1995. Blameless wrongdoing. *Ethics*, 106(1), pp. 120–127.

Tännsjö, T., 2010. *From reasons to norms.* Dordrecht: Springer.

2 Partiality and professional ethics in nursing care

This book concerns professional ethics regarding nursing care. I could also have used the terms 'nursing ethics', 'medical ethics', or 'health care ethics'. It is, however, presumably constructive to see the characteristic features of a profession in association with the questions of partiality and justice in nursing care. In fact, the underlying and divergent claims that form the debate between partial concerns and justice must be seen in the light of professional contexts. Nursing care has a more specific connotation than personal care, and my use of the term 'professional ethics' implies a particular approach. In the next section, I give a brief outline of some defining features of a profession. The account is based on Seumas Miller's (2010) teleological perspective of professions. Here I do not attempt to demonstrate that nursing in fact is a profession. My intention is rather to point to some features that characterise professions, which in turn can give us a clearer picture of the distinctiveness of the professional ethics of nursing care. Then I explore how the particular conceptualisation of professional roles influences our account of role morality and professional ethics. Based on Lawrence Blum's (1994) perspective on these issues, I will argue that the ethics of nursing is somewhere in between the merely personal and the merely impersonal. This brings us to a discussion of agent-relativity and partiality, which will be the topic for discussion at the end of this chapter.

Nurses and the nursing profession

> One of the strengths of an approach to professional roles which takes their moral status to depend importantly on their links with key human goods is that this sort of approach fits naturally with a central feature of any occupation's claim to be a profession in the first place. That is, it is widely agreed that for an occupation justifiably to claim to be profession, its practitioners must deal not simply with goods that many of us strongly desire to have; rather its practitioners must be able to help us attain certain goods that play a crucial strategic role in our living a flourishing life for a human being.
>
> (Oakley and Cocking, 2001, p. 79)

Being constituted by institutional rights and duties that are also moral rights and duties is one defining characteristic of a profession (Miller, 2010). Some of these rights and duties are special in that people outside the profession are not obligated by the same set of values and duties (Miller, 2010; Grimen, 2008). Nurses, for instance, have a duty to provide proper and individualised nursing care for their patients. Members of other professions, such as teachers and lawyers, do not have this particular duty. There are at least two reasons for this. First, nursing care is based on the expert knowledge of the nursing profession. Some of this expert knowledge is to some degree also possessed by other professionals, such as physicians or members of other caring vocations like enrolled nurses, and by people in general. But the whole body of the particular expert knowledge of nursing is only possessed by members of the nursing profession. According to Miller (2010), the possession of expert knowledge is also another defining feature of a profession. Miller does not address what it takes to possess expert knowledge or what expert knowledge consists in other than, for example, medicine in the case of doctors. And he continues:

> If members of a profession, say, lawyers, are adequately to realize the ends of their profession (justice), then they need to possess expert technical knowledge (of the law). In contemporary societies this expert knowledge is in large part acquired by studying a degree at a university.
>
> (Miller, 2010, p. 182)

As for nurses, then, we could say that their expert knowledge is nursing, but that does not really tell us much. Nursing scholars have for decades discussed questions over what 'nursing' consists of and what it takes to possess it (Benner, 2000).[1] A frequently cited account of nursing knowledge is Carper's (1978) four patterns of knowledge in nursing. These are empirics (the science of nursing), aesthetics (the art of nursing), personal knowledge, and moral knowledge.[2] Although there is no single agreed upon definition of the body of knowledge in nursing, it incorporates knowledge both from theory and practice concerning patients' needs for medical treatment and nursing care.[3]

A second reason is that their social terms of reference ask nurses to pursue certain collective goods that members of other professions (nor people in general) do not pursue. According to Miller, the pursuit of certain collective goods is also a defining property of a profession. Miller defines collective goods as 'jointly produced goods that ought to be produced and made available to the whole community, because they are desirable goods and ones to which the members of the community have joint moral rights' (Miller, 2010, p. 75). The collective goods pursued by the nursing profession are represented by the four basic responsibilities of nursing: promoting health, preventing illness, restoring health, and alleviating suffering (The ICN Code of Ethics for Nurses, 2006). Although there is and has been some ambiguity concerning exactly what nursing is and consists of, I believe it is uncontroversial to claim that *care* with relation to the best interests of the sick or disabled individual is the basic virtue in any nursing activity. While care is a concept that it is notoriously hard to define in exact terms, nursing care is a specific form of caring which is initially focused on particular needs of the patient related to his or her health and medical condition. Providing individualised nursing care is one of the most important duties for a nurse. For the sake of convenience, and since there are a wide range of nursing care activities (some of them can be classified, others not), I refer to any such activity as a nursing project. It is important to note that a nurse has several nursing projects. For instance, some include dressing a wound, mobilising a frail patient, performing a morning toileting of a patient, communicating with a patient and his or her relatives, administering medications, assisting in medical procedures, etc. Or as Chambliss portrays it, '[c]lose patient contact, with all five senses, is nursing's speciality' (Chambliss, 1996, p. 64).

A nursing project[4] means any nursing activity that takes place in the encounter with individual patients, whether to promote health, to prevent illness, to restore health, or to alleviate suffering. This nursing-project sketch is central to my argument for partiality: that nurses might be permitted to act partially within the context and towards the purpose of carrying out their basic duties.

So far I have argued that their expert knowledge and the collective nature of their responsibilities means that nurses have special duties that are not required of other professionals. But another professional dimension of nursing is important to explore here – what Miller refers to as the professional–client relationship. Miller points to the distinction between market-based occupations, such as shopkeeping, and non-market-based occupations, such as the law or medicine. The former are characterised by a seller–buyer relationship where the economic purpose of making profit is the seller's main interest (Chambliss, 1996). Relationships in non-market-based occupations, on the other hand, are at least ideally not characterised by such concerns. For instance, in relationships between doctors and patients, economic concerns ought to be secondary to the needs of the patient and secondary to 'the requirement to provide the collective good definitive of the particular profession in question' (Miller, 2010, p. 181). Of particular interest here is the importance that Miller attaches to the precedence of the client's needs over commercial or other pressures in professional relationships (Miller, 2010, p. 181). Miller further emphasises the non-commercial basis of the professional–client relationship by pointing to the duty to care for clients as one of the fiduciary duties of non-market-based professions. As previously stated, care is a fundamental virtue in any nursing activity. And professional care is relational. To use the words of Chambliss, '[n]ursing care is hands-on, a face-to-face encounter with a patient' (Chambliss, 1996, p. 64), and 'to care for patients, then, first means that one works directly, spatially and temporally, with sick people' (Chambliss, 1996, p. 65). The problem of course is that claims of efficiency and maximising health-related benefits put pressure on nurses in their daily caring activities, especially when resources are scarce.

Now, to follow Miller, professional autonomy is a necessary precondition for pursuing the collective goods of the profession. Professional autonomy is a defining feature of professions, and it relates to decision-making and actions within the sphere of the profession (Miller, 2010). Professional autonomy needs special justification, which, Miller says, is provided by

> the (collective) ends of the professional role in question. Thus, surgeons ought to have professional autonomy just because this is the best way to maximise health of patients, given the expertise and knowledge possessed by surgeons (but not by nonsurgeons).
>
> (Miller, 2010, p. 187)

According to Miller's account, professional autonomy is exercised when (a) decisions and actions in question are 'his or her call' (Miller, 2010, p. 186), meaning he or she is the one to make the decision, and (b) the decision cannot be overridden by a superior (Miller, 2010). As Miller argues, '[a] surgeon, for example, has to make a decision as to whether to operate, a decision that cannot be overridden by a hospital administrator' (Miller, 2010, p. 186). But whether professional autonomy can be exercised properly according to these principles is questionable. Oftentimes other, non-professional concerns will challenge and limit professional autonomy. The surgeon in Miller's example cannot base his or her decision solely on medical concerns, but also has to take into account, for instance, health care policies with regard to priority setting, budgets, and efficiency claims. Additionally, the patient's own autonomy must be taken into account in particular situations. Nurses have even less autonomy over their own organisation and practice than do physicians, since nurses also assist in medical treatment ordered and controlled by physicians. This situation is probably most evident in nursing care in hospitals, whereas, for instance, public health nurses and midwives possess greater agency to exercise autonomy. Nevertheless, autonomy functions at the very least as an ideal in many professions. Moreover, since, as I will argue, partiality might actually serve to protect the nursing project, nurses' autonomy in deciding how and what to prioritise is an important dimension of this idea.

It is noteworthy that professional autonomy coheres with professional liability and discretion. As Miller notes, 'if members of a profession are adequately to realise the ends of their profession, they also need to possess a capacity to exercise discretionary judgment – including discretionary ethical judgment – in the application of their expert knowledge' (Miller, 2010, p. 182). Consequently, if nurses are to realise the goods of their profession, they also need to possess a capacity to exercise ethical judgment discretionally. This capacity to exercise discretionary judgment is an inevitable part of the profession's expert knowledge. With this in mind I maintain that the decisions and actions resting on professional moral responsibility to some degree depend on the individual nurse's comprehension of the values and ideals that inform nursing.[5] But even if nurses possess both autonomy and discretion, it does not necessarily follow that they have the ability to exercise it. As shown in the introduction, a nurse's ability to exercise autonomy and discretion is frequently constrained by lack of resources, as well as claims of efficiency and utility maximising.

The last feature of professions that Miller refers to is their institutionalisation. A person in a professional role is an institutionalised role occupant: 'Strictly speaking, the term profession refers to a set of such institutional-role occupants' (Miller, 2010, p. 182). A central point here is that professionals relate to the institution through which they undertake their roles. At the same time professional bodies or associations also form a kind of social institution. In Miller's words,

> doctors undertake their professional roles in the context of a health care system, comprised as it is of hospitals, surgeries, medical laboratories, and so on. Moreover, members of the professions are members of a professional body that is itself an institution, for instance, the American Medical Association …
>
> (Miller, 2010, p. 182)

Although it is commonly held that nurses, like other professionals, are institutional role occupants, these are not roles in a narrow sense of the word. Or so I shall argue in the next section. I do also believe that the way we conceive of professional roles (here, the roles of nurses) does have implications for the way we explain and justify partiality as a normative consideration of professional ethics. Owing to the collective goods that nurses are expected to realise, professional ethical guidelines for nursing emphasise impartiality. These obligations and responsibilities of the nursing profession are general ones because they apply to any nurse (i.e. any occupant of the profession of nursing) (Nordhaug and Nortvedt, 2011). As we shall see in the following sections, such an account does not amount to pure agent-neutrality. And neither does it amount to agent-relativity, at least not in the ordinary meaning of the word.

Agent-relativity typically refers to reasons which are essentially personal in character. But personal, private preferences or relations should not take precedence in professional decision-making contexts. As Applbaum states, '[t]he professions characteristically put forth *role-relative* but *person-neutral* prescriptions' (Applbaum, 1999, p. 64). It is due time to consider these issues further. I shall base my discussion on Blum's account of vocational motivation and action. While Blum does not address the issue of professions per se, at least not unambiguously, I still find his arguments relevant to this discussion. Then later in this chapter, I explore in what way the reasons for partiality might relate to agent-relativity and agent-neutrality in nursing care.

Partiality and professional roles

While debates in the ethics literature about partiality and impartiality have mainly focused on dichotomising personal and impersonal relationships,

I will now focus on moral obligations arising from the specific roles assumed by professionals. Blum is one among a few writers who have focused on the relationship between care, partiality, and role obligations. In his essay 'Vocation, friendship, and community: limitations of the personal–impersonal framework' (Blum, 1994) he establishes his concept of roles from Dorothy Emmet's (1966) account of role morality. According to Emmet, professional roles and professional codes are the most articulated forms of role morality. Inspired by Talcott Parsons' account of professions,[6] Emmet's point of departure is that professions have a fiduciary trust to maintain certain standards of performance and competence to carry out functions valued in society (Emmet, 1966). Carrying out this professional role has to include professional integrity, and takes place in a relation to particular persons. Emmet terms the relation between the professional and the client as a *role relation*. This relation entails specific role obligations that sometimes overlap, but must be distinguished from personal obligations:

> As a directive of behaviour in certain kinds of relationship, it is structured by rules; if not by explicit and sanctioned rules, at least by implicit understandings, and maxims, or rules of thumb, as to how such a person would behave in this kind of relationship.
>
> (Emmet, 1966, p. 158)

Professional codes, Emmet says, can be

> justified on functional grounds, as promoting the kind of relationship within which a job is most likely to be done effectively. But its importance is not only functional; the behaviour becomes valued on its own account as a matter of professional integrity, and adds to the respect with which a professional person is regarded in the community.
>
> (Emmet, 1966, p. 162)

From this, Emmet's conception of role involves the imposition of a specific set of obligations on the person who occupies the role. This set of obligations applies to anyone occupying that role, but not to those who do not occupy that role. The 'role morality' in this sense is general, but not universal. Besides, it is according to Blum, not wholly impersonal in the 'view-from-nowhere' sense, because of the historical contingencies bound up with moralities in particular societies (Blum, 1994, p. 103). Because of this, it is highly unlikely that the existence of a specific role with its responsibilities is derived directly from a pure impersonal point of view, says Blum (1994, p. 103). Role morality is impersonal only in the sense that it applies to *any* occupant of the role in question, i.e. it is externally placed on that role occupant independently of personal characteristics of that person, says Blum (1994). Actions taken based on role responsibility in this sense are therefore distinct from both personal and impersonal action.

According to Blum, then, those writers dealing with the conflict between personal and impersonal projects make the assumption that ethical reflection takes place within a framework solely defined as a personal–impersonal dichotomy. Against the moral psychology implied in the personal–impersonal framework, Blum argues that there is a large range of types of action and motivation that fall neither on the side of the personal nor one the side of the purely impersonal. One of these types of action stems from one's understanding of one's vocation. According to Blum, vocational action can take on a character that is more or less impersonal as well as a more or less individual and particularistic. In what follows, my aim is to explore how Blum's account of vocational motivation and action might be a valuable contribution to the discussion of partiality in nursing care.

Blum's argument is based on an example from Herbert Kohl's book *Growing Minds: On Becoming a Teacher* from 1984. While Blum does not explicitly use the word 'partiality' in his discussions of vocational acts and motivations, the following example is a case in point of my discussion of the topic:

> Kohl, then a secondary school teacher, was asked by some parents in a school in which he was teaching if he could give special tutoring to their son. The boy was 14 years old and did not know how to read. He was a large boy, angry and defiant; his teachers did not know how to handle him. Kohl agreed to work with the boy two days a week after class. Kohl worked with the boy for several months. He found him extremely difficult and never grew to like him personally. But eventually he helped the boy to begin reading. Kohl describes how he came to take a personal interest in the boy's progress as a learner and to find satisfaction in what the boy was able to accomplish under his tutelage.
>
> (Blum, 1994, p. 101)

As defined previously, partiality as part of nursing care means that where relational proximity prevails a patient's nursing care needs might be given precedence over other patients' needs. In the case of teaching, we could use a similar definition: Partiality as part of teaching means that in the presence of relational proximity a pupil's tutoring needs might take precedence over other pupils' tutoring needs. Admittedly, the text does not tell us whether this special tutoring in fact took *precedence* over other pupils' needs. What we do know is that Kohl spent some extra time and energy on one particular pupil, not on other pupils. Consequently, it might be the case that other pupils could also have benefited, some perhaps more so, from Kohl's special tutoring. And even more importantly, other pupils could have had greater needs for special tutoring than did this boy. The special tutoring two days a week for several months was given to one out of many pupils. Indeed, this is a case of favouring one person's needs.

According to Blum, Kohl's choice to provide extra tutoring to one student was not motivated by personal reasons. Kohl's motivation was not to promote his personal benefit or self-realisation, in fact, the request for tutoring may even have been inconvenient for Kohl. And, noteworthily, the fact that Kohl happened to not like the boy very much probably made it an unenjoyable experience for him. This latter point is worth emphasising because Kohl's choice to go ahead with the tutoring, which might be considered (as Blum does) a part of his role responsibility, also illustrates that these kinds of actions and forms of partiality can be independent of personal relationship or preferences between the parties involved. Neither do Kohl's actions fall under impersonal moral demands; as Blum says, there was no obligation, no requirement to help the boy, and the teacher did not experience an obligation or requirement to do so. In some sense, this special concern seems akin to supererogation. Let me pause with this for a moment. My approach to justify partiality in nursing care does not initially concern supererogatory acts – on the contrary. What I will argue later in this book is that partiality might be permissible as a means to providing nursing care. Supererogatory acts represent a different moral category than that of permissibility or require-ments. A quite common comprehension of supererogatory acts is formulated by Dancy:

> Supererogatory acts are those which lie 'above and beyond the call of duty'. Such acts characteristically enjoy a very high degree of value, probably more value than any other act available to the agent. But in thinking of them as supererogatory, we are thinking of them as actions which it is not wrong of the agent not to do.
>
> (Dancy, 1993, p. 127)

Hence, if partiality is equivalent to supererogation in nursing care, we limit it to nursing care activities that are good to do, but not those where it is bad when they are not done. Perhaps activities such as spending one's spare time at work voluntarily caring for one of the patients at the ward would qualify as partiality in a supererogatory sense. It would presumably be a good thing to do, but not a bad thing not to do. But of consideration here is partiality as a prerequisite for discharging nurses' responsibilities. Since supererogation is to do something 'extra', beyond one's obligations and responsibilities, it should not be a problematic instance of partiality.

That being said, let us continue to explore Blum's analysis of this example. Blum continues by arguing that Kohl's act was not motivated by an impersonal 'view-from-nowhere' perspective.

Rather, Blum writes, '[Kohl] responded to, was moved by, the particular boy's plight, namely his being 14 years old and unable to read' (1994, p. 102).

Kohl responded to a particular person and this person's particular needs. As for the question of partiality, Kohl did not (necessarily) have a pre-existing partial standing towards this boy. Kohl's motivation (for acting partially) was not presupposed by a relationship between him and the boy (or his parents). His actions were motivated by something else. But it was not, to follow Blum, motivated by an impersonally derived value that generated a reason for all to do the same thing in a similar situation. It is essential to notice that Kohl did not act *simply* as person concerned about the boy; Kohl acted *as a teacher*. The motivational force stems from Kohl's understanding of his professional values and responsibilities. As a teacher confronted by the boy's plight, Kohl decided to act as he did. On Miller's (2010) account, he is pursuing the collective good of the teaching profession by the use of his expert knowledge. Additionally, it seems obvious that he exercised ethical discretion combined with professional autonomy. One might also suppose that the relationship between him and the boy took precedence over any economic interest – though, indeed, the example does not mention if Kohl was paid by the parents.

This example is very similar to many of the moral dilemmas that arise in clinical nursing (and medicine for that matter). There are many instances in nursing when one responds to a patient's situational plight, as one hurries to a patient with respiratory distress or severe and acute instances of pain. In such situations one responds empathically and spontaneously, as a nurse with the particular knowledge and competency, along with the moral principles of benevolence and acute care that guide the nursing profession. It is interesting that a motivation may be seen as partialist in the sense that it is situational and particularistic. One does not respond to the patient's acute needs simply because it is the right thing to do according to universal principles; the motivation is also situational in so far as it is driven by empathic affective responses to the suffering of another.[7] But we should understand this empathic affective response as part of a professional recognition of the situation at hand. This has to do with the nurse's understanding of the values of the nursing profession, combined with their expert knowledge. The professional response in these examples is neither purely personal nor purely impersonal.

Now, in Emmet's account of roles, to occupy a role is to have a job description. But Kohl did not have a role obligation (in Emmet's understanding of the concept) to help the boy. As mentioned earlier, Kohl did pursue the collective good of his profession, but the *act in question* (extra tutoring) did not result from a specific role responsibility or job description. The role of a teacher is a richer concept than Emmet's use of the term 'role', and is, according to Blum, an example of a vocation. It invokes a general place and purpose in society and carries with it certain values, standards, and ideals, Blum says. At this point the distinction between roles and vocation becomes more evident. Moreover, since a paradigm vocation, according to Blum, is one that both realises excellences and serves a good end or ends (not necessarily moral ends), I think one can also say that the distinction between roles and professions becomes more evident. Before I continue, we should observe that the notion of vocation can have different meanings: It can be understood as a calling or as a profession. Blum's intended connotation appears somewhat ambiguous at this point. To the extent that this is an important distinction to make, my strategy is to suggest that Blum's concept of vocations is closest to that of professions. Nevertheless, being a professional can also be a calling, but that fact does not influence the argument.

Since roles (in Emmet's sense of the term) are like job descriptions, roles need not reflect the individual occupant's sense of personal value. A hallmark of a vocation is just such a reflection of the individual agent's understanding of the values and ideals of his or her vocation (Blum, 1994). According to Blum's argument, this individual understanding and comprehension of values and ideals generates what the agent experiences as moral pulls. This means, for instance, in the case of Kohl, that another teacher may have a different interpretation of what teaching involves than does Kohl – and the same logic would apply to nursing as well. The insight from Blum here is that a personal identification with the values and ideals of one's profession (or vocation) is interwoven with the values and ideals of the profession in general.

The main difference between obligations from roles and obligations from vocation is, then, according to Blum, that the former is impersonal and external to the agent, whereas the latter is neither purely impersonal nor personal. Although this account so far seems reasonable to me, I find his arguments problematic at one point, particularly his account of the non-impersonal (personal) character of vocations: 'an individual with a vocation must believe deeply in the values and ideals of the vocation and must in some way choose or at least affirm them *for herself* (Blum, 1994, p. 104).

At first glance, this seems to me a far too demanding and perhaps also unreasonable claim. If a requirement of a vocation (or profession) is that those occupying it must experience a deeply *personal* identification with the values that inform the vocation in question, it follows that it might also exclude some persons in some situations. For instance, abortion or euthanasia might be controversial issues for some but not all health care professionals. Hence, in those countries where, for instance, euthanasia is a legal practice, those physicians who find this practice immoral may not want to choose that particular vocation. But this is probably a misconstruction of Blum's argument. For one thing, Blum's point is that one's vocation is constitutive of one's identity and moral orientation (at least for a certain period of one's life). In other words, one perceives the values and responsibilities of one's vocation because of one's values (Blum, 1994).

In such an interpretation lies a danger of arbitrariness. But at the same time, there is a way vocational action can be said to be impersonal, in that it is a response to something external and objective (Blum, 1994). Let me present one more citation from Blum that I think captures the essence of his account:

> The vocational agent does not take herself to be pursuing a goal simply because of its value to *her*. It is not *because it is part of her project* that she is impelled to help the pupil, to give extra tutoring to the student, and the like. Rather, the vocational agent takes herself to be responding to a value outside of herself, following (what she takes to be) its dictates. She

is not pursuing a merely personal value either in the sense of something unconnected with the claims of other persons or the sense in which she sees the reason for its pursuit as being conferred by its place in her own personal goals.

(Blum, 1994, p. 106)

A final point worth emphasising is that caring represents a fundamental dimension of vocations. According to Blum, there is a significant way in which caring in vocations has a wider scope than merely the fulfilment of a role.

Hence, to be caring, the professional's concern must involve some regard for the patient's overall good (but it is not all-embracing as it is in parent-hood) and a sense of how the good of the activity fits into the receiver's overall good (Blum, 1994). This is also very well exemplified in nursing. As a nurse one is not simply motivated by patients as a deeply personal value, as a project for oneself as a private person. Motivations in nursing care are orchestrated by values of benevolence and non-harming as well as doing what is best for the patient. At the same time, it is significant that the ideals of benevolence in medicine and nursing and doing the best for one's patient are partialist in some very distinct sense. The sense of commitment arising from such an understanding of one's professional role cannot be seen as separate from situations in which partiality might be permissible. In relational proximity to the sick and needy patient, this commitment becomes even more evident. It is a partialist principle of giving priority to one's patient or the patients under one's duty that has for centuries guided the medical as well as other health care professions (Tranøy, 2005). Partiality based on one's understanding of one's profession resembles a particularistic motivation central to nursing care. Conceptualising nursing as a professional role, or vocation, will engender certain commitments to patients that are neither personal nor private in the more intimate sense. But neither are they impersonal in the strictly objective sense, as obligations and rules externally placed upon a nurse. Hence, the special obligations of nursing as a professional role will throw new light on the relationship between partial and impartial moral demands. In particular, it will enrich the traditional notion of partiality as something belonging only to the domain of private and personal morality, having less impact on larger societal obligations.

Partiality, agent-relativity, and agent-neutrality

Although the reasons for impartiality are often used synonymously with agent-neutrality, and the reasons for partiality are often used synonymously with agent-relativity (Feltham, 2010), this assumed correspondence lacks an underlying connection. I have already indicated that reasons for partiality in nursing care are role-relative, which can be taken to mean that they are nei-ther purely agent-neutral nor agent-relative. In this section, I will explore the connections between these concepts and partiality. Then in Chapter 5 I return to the issue of agent-centredness in advancing an argument for a prerogative for partiality in nursing care.

While underscoring the lack of a single, agreed upon definition of these terms, Feltham explains the basic difference between them as 'I have an agent-relative reason for action if my having that reason depends on something's being mine; while reasons that don't depend on such a relationship are agent-neutral' (Feltham, 2010, p. 3).

This argument may be hair-splitting, but this notion of 'something's being mine' is a bit puzzling regarding both agent-relativity and partiality. With regards to partiality in nursing care in particular, I think this notion might mislead us into taking an arbitrary or biased approach to partiality. I return to this in a few pages.

Why is this commonly used reference to *my* or *mine* slightly puzzling or even misleading? Obviously, a person who needs help does not have to be 'mine' for an agent-relative reason to come into play. More still, the reason applies to the agent; this is why it's called agent-relative, not 'appealer-relative' (or need-relative, or some other 'objective'-relative reason). The agent identifying with this reason can certainly explain this reason in terms of 'I have this reason because X is mine'. But the point about agent-relativity is not that X (for instance my daughter or my friend) is mine and that I should protect whatever or whomever *belongs* to me. The point is that the *reason* is mine because of some sort of *connection* between myself, what should or ought to be done, and the reason-giving person (or a characteristic about us, such as him being in need and I being the one able to meet this need). Another way of putting this is to say that an agent-relative reason is *only* related to the agent in question because of some characteristic of the *agent*. Take a look at the following example given by Raustøl:

> Consider, for instance, reasons to help Joe paint his house. One reason for helping Joe is that he would benefit. This reason does not depend on any special connection between Joe and the agent. So every agent has this reason. These reasons that do not depend on any special connection with the agent have come to be called *agent-neutral reasons*. But I have another reason for helping Joe, namely that he is my grandfather. This reason does depend on the special connection between the action of helping him and me, namely that he is my grandfather. And note that this reason necessarily refers back to me.
>
> (Raustøl, 2010, p. 17)

Here, the agent-relative reason (for helping one's grandfather) arises from the special connection between the agent (me) and the grandfather. It is the *relationship* between us that gives *me* a reason to help *him*.[8] Of course, helping one's grandfather does not necessarily entail partiality. But Raustøl uses this example to show that partialist reasons can be agent-relative.

This resembles an agent-relative, object-giving reason for partiality: I should help *grandfather*. But it could also be formulated as an agent-relative, subject-giving reason for partiality: *I (as a granddaughter and because I am the granddaughter) should help grandfather*. I return to object-giving and subject-giving answers to the question of partiality later in this section.

Now, as Raustøl opportunely remarks, there can also be agent-neutral reasons for partiality:

> For instance, if I hold that it is morally appropriate that we give more weight to the good of people who are badly off than people who are well off, then my view involves partiality. This view is a case of prioritarianism. However, I believe it is right that everyone should do this, not only I, or some. Furthermore, I believe that people should do this regardless of their connection with those who are badly off. So, the reason to act does not necessarily refer back to the agent: it applies equally to everyone. This is a case of *agent-neutral partiality*: it claims that everyone ought to give (some) special weight to the good of the worst off. Therefore, being partial is not necessarily the same as acting for an agent-relative reason.
>
> (Raustøl, 2010, p. 18)

Because agent-neutral partiality is focused on the needy and not on any particular agent, it resembles object-giving reasons for partiality. At first glance, agent-neutrality seems better fitted as the justificatory basis for partiality in nursing care: It is the patient, not the individual nurse, who is the centre of attention, and the reason for partiality stems from the patient *and* his or her need.

An agent-neutral reason is related to any agent, including the agent in question. An agent-neutral reason is therefore a universal reason. But it can also be a general reason, a reason for all those to whom the reason is relevant, for instance, a certain group of people. That is, anyone having a daughter has a general reason to care for his or her daughter. That is both an agent-relative reason for the agent in question and a general reason for any agent having a daughter. Analogously, I think we could say that a(ny) reason for partiality in professional contexts is a general role-relative reason, applying only to those occupying the profession. But it is not an agent-neutral reason in a 'view-from-nowhere' sense, to use Nagel's expression (Nagel, 1986). A situation in which care is involved should not be observed from the view from nowhere. It should be observed from the patient's perspective and through a professional and caring lens. Hence, the reasons for partiality that applies to nurses *as nurses* are role-relative. They are not agent-neutral in a universal sense since the reasons only apply to nurses, not to people in general (recall the special professional duties discussed earlier). Hence, we could call them role-relative. In particular, reasons for partiality in nursing care apply only to nurses since nurses provide nursing care. This is not to say that other health care professionals also might have similar reasons for partiality.

Another question is whether reasons for partiality in nursing care also can be agent-relative. In the discussion of Blum's account of professional role morality, I argued that there is an element of agent-relativity involved in partiality in nursing care. A central feature of professions (or vocations), as opposed to roles, is the importance of the agent's understanding of the values and ideals that inform the profession. This understanding is neither personal nor impersonal, but rather a hybrid of expert knowledge and role obligations integrated with the particularities of the patient's objective and subjective nursing care needs. So a central question of agent-relativity then is, as Feltham formulated it, 'whether I or some competent stranger should care for her' (Feltham, 2010, p. 3). Is the nurse replaceable to the patient? Given nurses' social terms of reference, the answer is no. That is, to use Miller's terms, nurses pursue some collective goods. And the pursuit of these collective goods (see the first section of this chapter) represents the social mandate of the nursing profession. From such a point of view, nurses are not replaceable to patients. But this does not really answer the question concerning agent-relativity. The question of interest would be whether a particular nurse is replaceable to this particular patient. Bubeck says that '[p]rivate role holders are hence unique and irreplaceable while public role holders are replaceable as long as they meet the requirements of the role' (Bubeck, 1995, p. 203). But of course, this is an empirical question. It seems plausible to assume that sometimes they are, sometimes they are not – depending on the individualities of both the nurse and the patient, as well as contextual circumstances. But since nursing care is directed to particular patients, but can only be performed by nurses, partiality must ascribe significance to both the patient and the nurse. That is, partiality cannot be considered exclusively from the agent's perspective; it is other-oriented. Partiality in nursing is a form of altruism since, as De Gaynesford (2010) points to, the term places no special emphasis on the agent, but labels a preference or particular concern for certain others.

This also resembles Blum's definition of altruism: 'By "altruism" I will mean a regard for the good of another person for his own sake, or conduct motivated by such regard' (Blum, 1980, p. 10). Benevolence is a fundamental part of altruism, but any connotation of self-sacrifice or self-neglect is not a part of this concept: '[T]o say that an act is altruistic is only to say that it involves and is motivated by a genuine regard for another's welfare; it is not to say that in performing it the agent neglects his own interests and desires' (Blum, 1980, p. 10).

This pertains to both an object-giving answer and a subject-giving answer to the question: '[W]hy [what reasons do you have to] practice a preferential option for x?' (De Gaynesford, 2010, p. 95). De Gaynesford distinguishes between two categories of object-giving answers to this question:

1   Other-object: e.g. because x is *poor*; or x is *English*; or x is *female* (i.e. a preferential option for the poor, the English, women).
2   Self-object: i.e. because x is *one's own* (in some way) – i.e. first-personal partiality (each agent will translate the principle for themselves as 'because x is *mine* [or ours]')

(De Gaynesford, 2010, p. 95)

From this we obtain the following two object-giving answers to the question of why should a nurse practise partiality to a certain patient:

(1a)   Other-other: e.g. because the patient here and now is in need of nursing care (i.e. partiality towards present persons in need of nursing care).
(2a)   Subject-object: i.e. because it is the nurse's patient (in some way) – i.e. first-person partiality.

De Gaynesford offers, then, two categories of subject-giving answers to the question: 'Who practices a preferential option for x?':

3   Other-including-subject: one does/one should (depending on the normative status of the reason).
4   Other-excluding-subject: I do/I should (depending on the normative status of the reason).

(De Gaynesford, 2010, p. 95)

From this, we can establish two categories of subject-giving answers to the question: '[W]ho practises partiality towards a particular patient?':

(3a)   Other-including-subject: Any nurse does/should.
(4a)   Other-excluding-subject: I (as a nurse) do/should.

By cross-categorising, De Gaynesford says, we then obtain (for the case of 'should' rather than 'do'):

a   One should because x is poor
b   I should because x is poor
c   One should because x is one's own
d   I should because x is mine

(De Gaynesford, 2010, pp. 95–96)

In the case of nursing, we then obtain:

(a$_1$)   Any nurse should because the patient here and now is in need of nursing care.
(b$_1$)   I (as a nurse) should because the patient here and now is in need of nursing care.
(c$_1$)   Any nurse should because it is the nurse's patient (in some way).
(d$_1$)   I (as a nurse) should because the patient is mine.

Whereas (a_1) arises due to characteristics about the patient (i.e. he or she is a present patient in need of nursing care), (c_1) is focused on the agent. In any of these cases, these reasons point back to any nurse (and only nurses). Both (a_1) and (c_1) represent general role-relative reasons for partiality. This means that any nurse, but not any person in general, could have these reasons. Hence, this is not agent-neutrality in an impersonal and universal sense; the agent has to be a nurse, and the reason has to refer back to *any* nurse. Both (b_1) and (d_1) are also role-relative reasons, but they appeal to individual nurses in particular cases. In this case (b_1) is focused on the patient, and (d_1) is focused on the agent. Hence, we have both object-giving and subject-giving reasons that are role-relative, either formulated in general terms or directed at individual nurses. But notably, these are not agent-relative reasons in the personal sense. It is only *because I am a nurse* that I have these reasons. Suppose, for instance, that my friend is hospitalised because she needs an infusion of antibiotics. Do I have an agent-relative reason for administering antibiotics to my friend? I certainly have a reason for doing the best I can to comfort her and so on. But I do not have a reason for administering her medications unless, and this is my point, I am the nurse responsible for this patient. Then the reason applies to me as the agent, but not to me as a private person. This is why I prefer to use the term 'role-relative'. Role-relative reasons, then, include elements both from agent-relativity and agent-neutrality but are fundamentally tied to a certain profession.

Now, at the beginning of this chapter, I said that an argument based on 'something being mine' might mislead us into accepting arbitrary or biased approaches to partiality in nursing care. As I noted in the introduction, partiality based on personal preferences or pre-existing bonds between the nurse and the patient is clearly problematic. But still, reasons for partiality arise basically from the encounter with the needy patient here and now, regardless of an identification of the patient as 'mine'. The focus is on the patient, not on the nurse. Nevertheless, I will emphasise the importance of (to some extent) particularistic concerns that allow for nurses to make subjective choices (compare the discussion of Blum's account of professions/vocations). This is crucial, for as I already have alluded to, professional commitments may include various ways of behaving partially that are essential to practices of caring, and which also might throw altogether new light on the partialist–impartialist debate.

To sum up, then, I have argued that reasons for partiality arise from the connection between the nurse and the patient. These reasons are either general role-relative reasons (a reason for any nurse) or they can be taken to be particular role-relative reasons – i.e. applying to me *as a nurse* here and now. In both cases, reasons can point back to both the patient (object-giving reason) and/or the nurse (subject-giving reasons). In any of these cases, nurses are also obligated according to some impartial concerns. The question is, of course, where the limits between concerns for partiality and concerns for impartiality should be drawn. This question will be the subject of discussion in Chapters 5 and 6.

Concluding remarks

This chapter has focused on professional ethics and partiality. I have outlined how nursing should be understood as a professional role distinct from other contractual role-occupations in a way that influences the way role morality is comprehended. Nursing involves ethical concerns fusing the impartial and the partial. As members of the nursing profession, any nurse possesses responsibility for pursuing certain collective goods that should be distributed fairly. These goods are represented by the four clinical concerns of promoting health, preventing illness, restoring health, and alleviating suffering. Any caring activity falls under at least one of these areas of responsibility. Nursing care is based on a sensitivity to the particularities of specific situations, awareness of patients' needs, as well as the actual performance of the relevant caring services. Since caring services take place in the encounter with the patient, they require some degree of time and attention with regard to the particular patient. Individualised nursing care is one of the most important duties and responsibilities of nursing, and can be articulated in terms of role-relativity. But as part of prioritising, partiality might sometimes be important for providing individualised nursing care, i.e. in order to fulfil particular nursing projects. Still, a further normative justification of partiality is needed. In Chapter 5 I will aim to advance such an argument. But in the meantime: Given the central role that needs assessments play for the discussion on partiality and justice in nursing care, the next chapter will explore the complexities relating to identifying and classifying needs.

Notes

1 See for instance Meleis (2012).
2 White (1995) has suggested an additional pattern: the sociopolitical, which is knowledge about the context of nursing.
3 This includes for instance knowledge gained from practical experience, tacit knowledge, ethical knowledge, theoretical knowledge from nursing science and research, as well as scientific knowledge from other professions such as medicine, sociology, and psychology.
4 Note that I am only concerned about clinical nursing care. My arguments in this book are not aimed at nursing activities taking place in other areas or levels of health care, such as health-care administration.
5 More on this is given in the next section.
6 See, for instance, ch. 10: 'Social structure and dynamic process: The case of modern medical practice', in Parsons (1951). From the perspective of Emmet's usage, the most interesting is the emphasis Parsons places on the *instrumental and functional roles* of both the doctor and the patient. The relationship between the professional and the client is an instrumental relationship where different normative role-expectations play a significant part in the interactions between the role-takers.
7 See for instance Nortvedt (2012) and Nortvedt and Nordhaug (2008).
8 One could ask whether a particular agent-relative reason just applies to one agent, or whether several agents have this very same agent-relative reason. Suppose that my grandfather needs help painting his house, and I have an agent-relative reason to help him because he is my grandfather. But is this reason only mine or does the very same reason apply to my brother and my cousins of whom my grandfather is also their grandfather?

References

Applbaum, A., 1999. *Ethics for adversaries: The morality of roles in public and professional life*. Princeton, NJ: Princeton University Press.

Benner, P., 2000. *From novice to expert: Excellence and power in clinical nursing practice, commemorative edition*. Englewood Cliffs, NJ: Prentice Hall.

Blum, L., 1980. *Friendship, altruism and morality*. London: Routledge & Kegan Paul.

Blum, L., 1994. *Moral perception and particularity*. Cambridge: Cambridge University Press.

Bubeck, D., 1995. *Care, gender, and justice*. Oxford: Clarendon Press.

Carper, B., 1978. Fundamental patterns of knowing in nursing. *Advances in Nursing Science*, 1(1), pp. 13–23.

Chambliss, D., 1996. *Beyond caring: Hospitals, nurses, and the social organization of ethics*. Chicago: University of Chicago Press.

Dancy, J., 1993. *Moral reasons*. Oxford: Blackwell.

De Gaynesford, M., 2010. The bishop, the valet, the wife, and the ass: What difference does it make if something is mine? In: Feltham, B. and Cottingham, J., eds, *Partiality and impartiality: Morality, special relationships, and the wider world*. Oxford: Oxford University Press, pp. 84–97.

Emmet, D., 1966. *Rules, roles and relations*. London: Macmillan.

Feltham, B., 2010. Introduction: Partiality and impartiality in ethics. In: Feltham, B. and Cottingham, J., eds, *Partiality and impartiality: Morality, special relationships, and the wider world*. Oxford: Oxford University Press, pp. pp. 1–25.

Grimen, H., 2008. Profesjon og profesjonsmoral. In: Molander, A. and Terum, L., eds, *Profesjonsstudier*. Oslo: Universitetsforlaget [Norwegian], pp. 144–161.

Meleis, A., 2012. *Theoretical nursing: Development and progress*. 5th edn. Philadelphia, PA: Lippincott Williams and Wilkins.

Miller, S., 2010. *The moral foundations of social institutions: A philosophical study*. Cambridge: Cambridge University Press.

Nagel, T., 1970. *The posibility of altruism*. Princeton, NJ: Princeton University Press.

Nagel, T., 1986. *The view from nowhere*. New York: New York University Press.

Nordhaug, M. and Nortvedt, P., 2011. Justice and proximity: Problems for an ethics of care. *Health Care Analysis*, 19, pp. 3–14.

Nortvedt, P., 2012. The normativity of clinical health care: Perspectives on moral realism. *Journal of Medicine and Philosophy*, 37(3), pp. 295–309.

Nortvedt, P. and Nordhaug, M., 2008. The principle and problem of proximity in ethics. *Journal of Medical Ethics*, 34(3), pp. 156–161.

Oakley, J. and Cocking, D., 2001. *Virtue ethics and professional roles*. Cambridge: Cambridge University Press.

Parfit, D., 1984. *Reasons and persons*. Oxford: Clarendon Press.

Parsons, T. 1951. *The social system*. London: Routledge.

Pettit, P., 1987. Universalizability without utilitarianism. *Mind*, 96(381), pp. 74–82.

Raustøl, A., 2010. Impartiality and partiality in nursing ethics. s. 1. Dissertation, University of Reading.

The ICN Code of Ethics for Nurses, 2006. www.icn.ch/images/stories/documents/about/icncode_english.pdf [Accessed 14 July 2012].

Tranøy, K., 2005. *Medisinsk etikk i vår tid*. Bergen: Fagbokforlaget [Norwegian].

White, J., 1995. Patterns of knowing: Review, critique, and update. *Advances in Nursing Science*, 17(4), pp. 73–86.

3   On the concept of need for nursing care

This chapter is devoted to an analysis of the need concept as it relates to nursing care. It may, however, be difficult to give a precise definition of this concept. For one, the concept is not permanent or static; it is, rather, influenced by culture and history, and its meaning has changed over time. For instance, in the 1950s there were debates concerning whether parents should be allowed close contact with their hospitalised children. Some argued that close contact between parents and hospitalised children was psychologically detrimental for the child. Today, it is generally accepted that hospitalised children need close contact with their parents, siblings, and so on.

The concept of need for nursing care can also, as we shall see, be relative to a patient's own experiences and perceptions. Moreover, the concept may have different connotations and is sometimes difficult to distinguish from mere desires. For instance, a patient saying 'I need something to drink' may express the subjective need of feeling thirsty. While this may be a result of dehydration, it might also express a mere desire for something pleasant, for example a desire for a glass of wine. If that is the case, it need not qualify as a need for nursing care at all.[1]

That said, the vast majority of substantial needs for nursing care probably are legitimate. Still, not all such needs are equally demanding, nor equally pressing. Besides, needs can be hard to identify and classify because of their complexity, and they can be difficult to compare when resources must be allocated between patients. Due to the complexities concerning the relations or distinctions between objective and subjective needs, and patients' co-morbidity, it proves difficult to subsume any need for nursing care under a comprehensive system of classification, both conceptually and substantially. But for the purpose of coming to terms with needs assessments in nursing care, we can make use of three categories of needs: (a) vital needs, (b) needs related to preventing or alleviating harm and suffering, and (c) needs related to flourishing and well-being.[2] In other words, if nursing care needs are going unmet, a patient either cannot live, cannot flourish, might be harmed, or continues to suffer. All these categories of needs have normative importance in nursing care and relate in one way or another to the four basic areas of nursing responsibility: promoting health, preventing illness, restoring health, and alleviating suffering.[3]

This chapter does not aim to define needs in more or less exact terms, i.e. delineating 'what it is and what it isn't'. Besides, as will be illustrated, the complexities relating to identifying and classifying needs influence the way nursing care needs should be conceptualised. For the most part, the discussion in this chapter is based on Soran Reader's (2007) account of needs as fundamental to normative ethics. Although Reader does not explicitly speak about professional practices, her account is taken to be a valuable contribution especially to the way we conceive of the normative importance of the concept of need in nursing practices. The chapter starts out with a discussion of two claims regarding features of the need concept and the relevance of these claims for the ways needs are conceived of in practice. The first feature concerns the distinctions between objective needs, subjective needs, and desires. As will be shown, these distinctions may be a useful analytical tool for identifying and classifying needs, but it may be unclear in clinical practice.

The second central feature relates to Reader's claim that needs statements are bidirectional. On one hand, a needs statement articulates what is morally demanding by stating what is missing, i.e. what the person in need lacks or is about to lack. On the other hand, a needs statement dictates what should be done to satisfy this demand (Reader, 2007). When exploring this claim in the context of nursing care, it becomes evident that needs statements are far more complex than this. At a conceptual level, this complexity relates to the distinctions between objective needs, subjective needs, and desires. But it also relates to the substantial complexities of patients' co-morbidity, capacity of comprehension and articulation, and autonomy, as well as the varieties of nursing care approaches for satisfying needs.

After reviewing these features, a rather brief outline of some normative implications will be discussed. The last two sections explore and discuss the moral demandingness of needs for nursing care. This relates to discussions concerning the extent to which needs must be occurrent to be morally demanding, and the idea that needs are presented as moral demands in the context of a relationship with an agent.

Before the central features of the need concept and its normative implications are discussed, some preliminary remarks about the need concept are given. This is to clarify what *kinds* of needs nursing care deals with. Additionally, some of the complexities involved in needs assessments are illustrated.

Central features of the needs concept

In order to come to terms with the rather wide concept of need, we require an analytical tool to distinguish the different categories of needs. In the following I will make use of Reader's analysis of the moral demandingness of needs by discussing her main arguments for a needs-based account of ethical practice. The chapter starts out with Reader's two claims related to central features of the needs concept. The first feature regards the claim that needs are objective and therefore non-intentional. The second claim for discussion is that needs statements are bi-directional. I review these arguments successively and discuss them in light of nursing care.

Needs and desires

Reader's first claim is that the needs concept refers to something objective. This means that needs, as contrasted to desires, are non-intentional. Non-intentionality should here be taken to imply that needing something is not dependent on 'the working of one's mind', i.e. being consciously aware of one's need. Instead, it depends on the way things really are (Wiggins and Dermen, 1987): 'I can only need to have x if whatever may be identical with x is something that I need' (Wiggins and Dermen, 1987, p. 62).

From this, we could say that in nursing care (a) a desire refers to that which the patient (consciously) wants – but not necessarily needs, whereas (b) a patient will be harmed or continue suffering, or not be able to flourish, or not able to live if a *need* is unmet. But a need is not *necessarily* something one wants or desires, or even is aware of. The statement that the needs concept refers to something objective is important, although complicating, for the distinctions between objective needs, subjective needs, and desires. The relevance of this difference between a need and a desire may be important in needs assessments in clinical practice. But there is only a delicate distinction between what we could call subjective needs and desires. This is so because a desire may accompany a perceived need. And subjective needs play an important role in nursing care.

Analytically, we can distinguish between needs that are universal versus needs that are experienced subjectively and are related to an individual patient's personal perception of her medical situation and health condition. In the context of nursing care, universal needs are independent of the patient's cultural, historical background, but are basically common to any human being. Subjective needs, on the other hand, are not non-intentional, since they do depend – to some degree – on the 'working of the mind' of the patient. But they should nevertheless be considered legitimate needs for nursing care, in a conceptual sense, different from mere desires. This kind of subjectivity may be dependent on the patient's cultural, historical, social background, etc. The distinction between objective needs and subjective needs is often unclear in practice. Sometimes these needs overlap, i.e. they can entail many elements, they may be complex, and they may vary from individual to individual according to, for instance, age and co-morbidity. Besides, both objective needs and subjective needs can be more or less urgent, more or less grave. There is also a practical implication here concerning what kind of normative status these different concepts of needs should have.

As an illustration of these complexities, consider a patient with advanced cancer with a bad prognosis. Suppose there is a certain, very expensive medication that might extend his life for, say, one or two months. This may be of great – subjective – value for this particular patient (as well as his relatives and social network). The patient may therefore have a subjective need for this medication: To be confident that he 'tried everything', to spend more time with his nearest and dearest, to experience his daughter's wedding, or other things of importance for his well-being, his integrity, his quality of life, and so on. This (subjective) need may be urgent since time is running out. On the other hand, from the point of view of health care personnel, the need for this *particular* medication may not be seen as a (legitimate) objective need according to the patient's situation, side-effects and utility of the medication, and so on. But notably, the fact that this particular medication may not be considered an objective need from a professional point of view does not mean that the patient doesn't have an objective need for *some kind* of medical or nursing intervention. This is also an example of a conflict between the way needs are conceptualised and comprehended by health care professionals, and by the individual patient himself. One question then is what kind of normative status an articulated need for a *particular intervention* should have.

Consider then Wiggins and Dermen's formal definition of a need:

> I need [categorically] to have x
> if and only if
> I need [instrumentally] to have x if I am to avoid harm
> (Wiggins and Dermen, 1987, p. 64)

We could, in the context of nursing care, say 'if I am to live' or 'if I am to flourish'. In Wiggins and Dermen's definition of a need, the need is already identified and articulated in terms of what it would take to avoid harm (I need to have x). Such a definition may be analytically useful as a way of coming to terms with what a need really is. Yet as we have seen, identifying needs may be challenging in itself. And notably, there is another important distinction at play here. When we discuss the differences or relations between needs and desires, we should also be aware of the difference between (a) desiring something x_1 and needing something x_2, versus (b) – *being in the state* of either desiring something or actually needing something. In the latter case, the missing 'something' may not yet be identified. Hence, for the patient with cancer, he is obviously in the state of needing something. But it is not quite clear, and certainly not agreed upon, what this 'something' is. It might be the expensive medication, which is the patient's own expressed need. But from the point of view of health care workers, this 'something' may represent something else. With the best intentions and the best knowledge available concerning, for instance, the medication's unpleasant side-effects, they may argue that the patient actually needs something else, e.g. medication to alleviate physical and psychological pain. This problem is further addressed in the next section.

Let us consider another example probably more relevant in daily nursing care situations. Consider a patient saying 'I need something to drink'. The patient may be pleased when offered a glass of water. Or she may refuse it and require flavoured and carbonated water with ice cubes instead. The latter alternative is not necessarily an expression of a mere desire. But it may be a mere desire that is not particularly important for the patient's situation at all. If there is, for instance, no reason to think that the patient actually needs flavoured and carbonated water with ice cubes for her medical or health condition, but she simply prefers it to feel, say, extra comfortable, it may not qualify as a legitimate need requiring a particular nursing intervention. Note that this does not imply that the patient shouldn't have her preference obeyed, but it should not be given much priority either – as a desire offers opportunities, not demands, to act upon. But if, for example, this patient is suffering from severe nausea, and flavoured, carbonated water with ice cubes is the only thing she can accept then the request for flavoured and carbonated water with ice cubes is not only a desire, it is an expression of a subjective need – which in turn also meets (to some extent) her objective need for hydration.

These examples illustrate that the distinctions between desires and subjective needs may be difficult to comprehend in clinical practice. So far, we have seen that subjective needs relate to flourishing and well-being. It should, however, also be emphasised that both subjective and objective needs correspond with any of the three needs categories set out above. For instance, subjective needs may relate to vital needs, as when a patient, due to religious convictions, refuses life-saving treatment such as a blood transfusion. And objective needs may relate to needs concerning flourishing and well-being, such as, for instance, when nursing homes are facilitated for patients' privacy.

To summarise what has been said so far, there is no clear, empirically per-ceivable distinction between subjective needs and objective needs. However, conceptually, objective needs for nursing care could be described as needs that are universal and (empirically) observable, whereas subjective needs refer to an individual patient's personal perception of his medical situation and health condition. In this sense, only objective needs qualify as needs according to the premise of non-intentionality. Still, as has been argued, subjective needs for nursing care are of great importance for a patient's health condition. Therefore, objective needs and subjective needs both qualify as needs according the definition above: a need is something which, if left unmet, may result in the patient being harmed or continuing to suffer, or may lessen the patient's ability to flourish or even threaten his life. But the patient might not be consciously aware of the need, nor necessarily desire to have it met.

Needs statements

According to Reader, needs statements specify the helping action by high-lighting two issues. First, a needs statement emphasises that which the person in need lacks or is in imminent risk of lacking. Second, as when finding 'the missing piece', a needs statement points towards what should be done to restore that which is lacking. We should keep in mind that Reader here refers to a statement about an already identified need. In simple cases of unambiguity, this seems quite clear. For instance, the patient needs a glass of water to swallow his pills – give the patient a glass of water. But situations in nursing care are not always this uncomplicated. It might therefore be useful to distinguish between (a) a statement about what is needed, and (b) a statement about what kind(s) of intervention(s) or action(s) the agent should take to satisfy the need in an adequate way.

Imagine a patient who recently moved into a nursing home after suffering from a stroke. The patient has among other things lost her capacity to express herself verbally. Every morning when having breakfast, the patient starts crying quietly. What kind of need – or needs – relates to the fact that the patient is crying? Crying is an expression of a whole range of emotionally or physically painful conditions relating to the individual's situation. It is not, for instance, as simple as 'the patient is crying – make her stop crying', or 'the patient needs comfort – comfort her'. Often, needs related to nursing care are far too complicated to fit into a single description of a need. The patient's crying might be an expression of very different conditions, for instance, anger, grief, uncertainty about the future, physical pain, etc. What we have here, then, is a patient *in the state of needing something* relating to relief of physical or psychological pain or discomfort, or needing an improvement to her well-being. At this point, the need per se is not yet identified. The important point here is that, even if we can articulate a needs statement concerning what this patient's need is, it is not always obvious what the agent is to do about it.

Besides, sometimes, in situations where needs statements are quite easy to formulate, there may be more than one need present at the same time. Consider a severely ill patient suffering from an advanced stage of cancer with a bad prognosis. The patient develops a bacterial pneumonia. If the patient is to be cured of his pneumonia, he needs antibiotics. This is a vital need since pneumonia is a life-threatening condition for this patient. Suppose, then, that the patient refuses to receive the antibiotics, even though he consciously acknowledges that without the medication, his life expectancy would be severely and utterly reduced. So another needs statement here may be, 'This patient needs to have his autonomy respected – do not administer the antibiotic'. Is this a morally demanding need that should be respected? That depends, we could say, on many aspects of the situation. This raises both legal issues and matters of principle concerning a patient's right to refuse treatment and the health care personnel's duty to provide adequate and lifesaving treatment. But context-dependent and subjective needs should also be given due consideration. Sometimes, and perhaps quite often in clinical practice, needs and needs statements can conflict.

Despite the complexities concerning identification and statements of needs, the discussed features of the needs concept may serve as relevant, principal analytical tools in nursing care. In the next section two normative features of needs are discussed, both of which pertain to what could be termed a normativity of presence.

The normativity of presence

According to Reader, two conditions must be met for a need to represent a moral demand. For one thing, the need must be occurrent or about to be occurrent; and second, the person in need must be in a moral relationship with an agent. Unless these two conditions are satisfied, Reader says, acting upon the need is more or less optional. The rest of this chapter is devoted to discussing the resulting normative implications of this view for nursing care.

Occurrent needs and dispositional needs

We have seen that needs for nursing care regard patients' health and medical condition, and, if these needs are left unmet, the patient may be harmed or continue to suffer, lose his ability to flourish, or possibly even die. Any of these three categories of needs have normative importance in guiding nursing care. But obviously, they are not necessarily equally demanding nor equally pressing. Primarily, judgments of moral urgency involve assessments of severity and direness. For instance, the need for assistance in an emergency situation is no doubt more urgent than the need for assistance in teeth brushing. And obstructed breathing is more severe than a cold (everything else being equal). As already emphasised, however, needs for nursing care are not always suitable objects for such classifications and comparisons. This is particularly evident in areas of nursing practice where basic care is the focus of professional attention and responsibility. We should therefore aim for another approach for assessing and judging the (moral) urgency of needs for nursing care. What we are looking for is an account more relevant in all areas of nursing practice. One such approach, which is not primarily dependent on traditional classification according to severity and urgency, is Reader's differentiation between occurrent needs and dispositional needs: 'Occurrent needs are more urgent than dispositional ones by definition, because only in cases of occurrant needs does the needing being actually lack what it needs. It is this lack that actually obligates the moral agent to act' (Reader, 2007, p. 71).

Dispositional needs, Reader says, are needs we have simply by virtue of being who we are. For instance, 'I have a dispositional need for protection from harm, even when I am as safe as I could possibly be' (Reader, 2007, p. 71). But notably, a dispositional need represents a moral demand in situations where the need is about to become occurent.

The need for proper hydration of the human body may serve as a useful example for our discussion here. As a dispositional need it cannot be eliminated. Inspired by Reader's words, we could therefore say that I have a dispositional need for proper hydration, even when I am properly hydrated. This also means, for instance, that as long as my body is adequately hydrated, I might not be aware of it as a dispositional need. The need for proper hydration manifests itself when it becomes occurrent or is about to become occurrent. And that is when, according to Reader's account, the need for hydration actually obligates the agent. This means that a need for proper hydration obligates a nurse when (a) the need is occurrent, as for instance when the patient is, to some degree, dehydrated, or (b) the need is about to become occurrent, as for instance when the patient's condition increases the likelihood of dehydration.

How can this account of moral demandingness guide needs assessments in nursing care? It is clear that needs that are either occurrent or about to become occurrent are morally demanding for nurses. But nurses' responsibility as regards prevention of illness and suffering complicates the picture. Consider again the need for proper hydration. This need relates to any of the three categories of needs for nursing care. First and foremost, the need for proper hydration regards vital needs. Indeed, this may be a grave need, such as when a patient suffers from severe dehydration and loses consciousness. It that case, the patient's need for hydration is severe and urgent. But it may also be a less urgent and less grave need – here and now, relatively speaking – such as when a patient who undergoes chemotherapy is about to have diarrhoea. Diarrhoea is a frequent side effect of chemotherapy, often causing dehydration, which in turn may be a severe condition. It this latter case, the need for hydration is not, *here and now*, equally critical as in the case of the unconscious patient. Still, it is about to become occurrent, and should definitively obligate the nurse to response as to avoid *harm*. What, then, about the duty concerning prevention of illness or harm? As a dispositional need, the need for proper hydration cannot be eliminated. Due to their medical and health condition, many, if not all, patients are particularly vulnerable to changes in their hydration status. Preventing a need from becoming occurrent is therefore an important responsibility in nursing. Hence, in nursing care it is not only needs that are occurrent or about to become occurrent that are morally demanding. Indeed, prevention of a dispositional need from becoming occurrent is morally demanding, though perhaps not equally pressing.

Again, this relates to the sometimes-unclear distinction between objective and subjective needs. For instance, patients under intensive care sometimes experience severe thirst – even though they are (objectively) adequately hydrated. This illustrates that a subjective need (here, the experience of being thirsty) can be inconsistent with the sort of objective need *usually* associated with the expression of the very same need.[4] This is also true for the patient who says, 'I need something to drink'. This may be a quite urgent need if the patient feels thirsty and uncomfortable. In that case, the expression of her (subjective) discomfort is likely to correspond with her (objective) bodily need for hydration. But an expression of a need for water, for example, may also be an expression of a need for comfort or well-being. If that is the case, the need is occurrent and should, according to Reader's account, obligate the nurse to respond. But it is not necessarily a need that requires attention here and now. Hence, an occurrent need may be urgent, though not especially serious or grave at all.

To sum up so far, the following general contours of an account of moral urgency of nursing care needs emerge: Needs for nursing care are related to patients' health and medical condition, and, if left unmet, can lead to the harm or continued suffering of the patient, impair his ability to flourish, or threaten his life. Any of these three categories can be assessed according to severity and urgency. But for a need to represent a (pressing) moral demand, *here and now*, the need must be occurrent or about to become occurrent. A patient's need for well-being can therefore be more urgent than his vital needs, depending on the occurrence of the needs in question. This latter point seems quite simple and intuitive: The nurse is obligated to act in the presence of a need for nursing care. If we are to arrange needs for nursing care according to degrees of moral urgency – which was the aim of this section – the following claim seems plausible: As long as the need in question is occurrent or about to become occurrent, needs should be prioritised according to a hierarchy where vital needs are the most pressing, followed by needs related to harm and needs related to well-being. Additionally, dispositional needs for nursing care should be prevented from becoming occurrent.

Now, even though a need itself can be morally demanding, this is not sufficient, Reader says, for a need to *place* an actual moral demand on a particular agent. What is also required is that the patient is in a moral relationship with an agent. This last point is of particular importance for the rest of the argument in this book. It is important because it shows how proximity is a necessary tool, so to speak, for the nurse's ability to sensibly grasp (i) distinctions and relations between subjective needs and objective needs, (ii) distinctions between subjective needs and mere desires, (iii) the meaning of needs statements, and (iv) the degree of moral urgency of needs.

Encountering needs

> Only when their need is presented in relationship can it present an actual moral demand, just as only when someone asks a question can it present a demand for an answer.
>
> (Reader, 2007, p. 5)

So far we have seen that when a need is occurrent, or threatening to become occurrent, it represents a moral demand. But according to Reader, the need constitutes a *real* moral demand only when and in so far as the person in need is in a form of a moral relation to an agent. In other words, the patient's need constitutes a real moral demand only when and in so far as the patient is in a (moral) relation to a nurse. This could better be expressed the other way around: for a nurse to be obligated to respond to a patient's need, there must be a kind of encounter between the nurse and the patient.[5]

In order to clarify the normative implication of this claim, we should first make clear the notion of 'moral relation'. A way of explaining why we should consider nurse–patient relations as *moral* relations is by reference to patients' vulnerability and nurses' professional mandate.[6] A similar point is made by Gastmans: 'as vulnerable patients cannot meet their own needs, they must rely on the goodwill of caregivers, like nurses. Power imbalances in nurse–patient relationships contribute to patients' vulnerability and their reliance on nurses' goodwill not to harm them' (Gastmans, 2013, pp. 146–147).

So, given that nursing care is an ethical practice taking place in moral relations, we still need to clarify what is meant by the term 'relation'. According to Reader, a moral relationship can take many forms, but they share two defining features. First, it involves an actual connection, a real 'something between' agent and patient that links them together (Reader, 2007, p. 72). This 'something between' is a kind of contact or presence. Second, a moral relation must be epistemologically transparent. The premise of epistemological transparency implies that it must be possible for the agent to know about the person in need to whom the agent is related (Reader, 2007).

In the context of nursing care, we could say that a need is morally demanding for a (particular) nurse, under two conditions: The need must be occurrent or about to become occurrent, and the patient must be present (in some sense) for this (particular) nurse.

Notably, there can be many relationship forms qualifying as moral relationships of this kind. These 'actual connections' vary from short-term encounters to long-term relationships. An anaesthetic nurse taking care of a patient in the operating theatre, or a nurse encountering a patient in an emergency ward, are examples of the former kind of relation. Long-term relations are found, for instance, in rehabilitation units, nursing home wards, and long-term psychiatric wards.

Obviously, the moral urgency of needs must be seen in light of nurses' professional moral responsibility. As professional role occupants, nurses are committed to act according to their areas of responsibility.[7] This means, as stated in the Introduction of this book, that nurses ought to give due consideration to the needs of any patient. But the common feature of these moral relations, these real connections as defined here, is that this is where *nursing care actually can take place.* Hence, whereas nurses' professional responsibility is directed towards any patient in the first place, the professional commitment can only be acted upon in some kind of 'real connection' between nurse and patient. This point has importance for what shall be referred to as 'nursing projects'.

Concluding remarks

Obviously, since many needs can be present at the same time, the three identified categories of needs are not mutually exclusive. Besides, even though these categories are organised hierarchically according to severity of need, priority decisions in nursing care are far more complex than this. This is particularly evident in those areas of health care where daily priority decisions primarily concern basic care rather than more medically oriented nursing care activities for severely ill or injured patients. Moreover, a nurse ought to give priority to the most severe and urgent needs but is still committed to respond to other, less severe or less urgent needs. If we look at the examples given above on the complexities of formulating and assessing needs for nursing care, they point to another interesting but also problematic implication. If only needs that are unquestionable – or what we might call empirically observable and 'provable', so to speak – should be taken into account, a risk of paternalism is engendered. On the other hand, there is a risk of manipulation, arbitrariness, and unfair distribution of nursing resources if too much emphasis is put on subjective needs, especially coupled with vague limits regarding a patient's mere desires.

Many daily clinical priority decisions concern how to prioritise between needs at the equal 'level' of need, whether classified as objective or subjective. In those cases, the questions are how to prioritise between patients with relevantly equal needs concerning, for instance, well-being or needs relating to prevention of some kind of harm. These questions are particularly important for the discussion of partiality and justice in nursing care, and will be discussed more thoroughly in Chapter 6.

Concrete decisions in particular situations are often complex and require contextual sensitivity combined with professional knowledge concerning what is at stake and what should be done to help. The examples above point to the importance of contextual sensitivity and adequate time and attention for the nurse to be able to sensibly grasp what is at stake for the individual patient. In turn, this forms a significant base for an argument in support of partiality in nursing care. In the next chapter, I will aim to advance such an argument.

Notes

1 That depends, we could say, on the patient's situation as well as his medical and health condition.
2 For the sake of convenience, the terms 'flourishing' and 'well-being' are used interchangeably.
3 See Chapter 2.
4 The sensation of thirst is usually a sign of dehydration, but is also associated with some medications, treatments, and medical diagnoses.
5 See for instance Chapter 1.
6 See Chapter 2.
7 See Chapter 2, on nursing and the nursing profession.

References

Gastmans, C., 2013. Dignity-enhancing nursing care: A foundational ethical framework. *Nursing Ethics*, 20(2), pp. 142–149.

Reader, S., 2007. *Needs and moral necessity*. Abingdon: Routledge.

Wiggins, D. and Dermen, S., 1987. Needs, need, needing. *Journal of Medical Ethics*, 13, pp. 62–68.

4 Care ethics, partiality, and interpersonal relationships

In what way can partiality in nursing care be justified? The aim of Chapters 4 and 5 is to explore possible answers to this question. I will mainly build on two positions that hold relationships to be a source of moral responsibility – the care ethics approach and the relational duties and reasonable partiality approach. In this chapter I turn to the first of these approaches.

As a perspective that purports to defend the moral value of relational care, responsibility, and responsiveness towards the vulnerable person, care ethics is a central moral outlook in nursing care. Care ethics might therefore also be expected to advance arguments for partiality in other areas of professional care work (Nordhaug and Nortvedt, 2011a). Yet the main problem with care ethics is its ambiguity as a normative position. For instance, an ascription of moral value to relational care does not imply a justification for why we ought to act upon this moral value. In other words, it seems unclear how care ethics addresses what Korsgaard called the normative question: 'When we seek a philosophical foundation for morality we are not looking merely for an explanation of moral practices. We are asking what justifies the claims that morality makes on us' (Korsgaard, 1996, pp. 9–10). It is therefore important to further elaborate the normative consequences of such a relational conception of morality. In particular, for nursing it would be important to ascertain what such a moral conception would entail in different cases of moral conflicts (Nordhaug and Nortvedt, 2011a; 2011b; Nortvedt et al., 2011). In what follows, I shall explore these issues.

An ethics of care is a moral outlook that purports to defend the moral value of relational care, responsibility, and responsiveness *within* relationships. An ethics of care emphasises that the agent is responsible to actual persons to whom one relates, on the basis of the particular situatedness of the patient under care and not in accordance with abstract principles and conventions (Pettersen, 2008). The nursing profession has typically embraced care ethics: '[T]he nurse's experiences at the patient's bedside make the ethics of care seem especially plausible as the basic ethical model for nursing' (Andolsen, 2001, p. 41). Moreover, since what is central to an ethics of care is that relational caring entails a focus on the particularities and context of the relationships (Darwall, 1998), it is a central moral outlook for health care professionals in general.

In 1982, Carol Gilligan's book *In a Different Voice* (Gilligan, 1982) set the scene for the development of this moral perspective. Gilligan's book became an impetus for discussions on the relations between gender and moral thinking. Since the 1990s the literature and debates considering ethics of care have expanded rapidly. Today, three decades later, Gilligan's work is still the point of departure for debates on the conflicting claims of an ethics of care and an ethics of justice. The justice perspective of an ethics of care will be explored later in this chapter.

Although an ethics of care might be said not to constitute a fully developed moral theory, there are some major features among the variety of versions of this ethical approach. Virginia Held (2006) points out five characteristics. The first is its central focus 'on the compelling moral salience of attending to and meeting the needs of the particular others for whom we take responsibility' (Held, 2006, p. 10). Behind this is the recognition that every human being is dependent on care from the beginning of life, and that most of us will become ill and dependent at some point. Important in care ethics is that the moral claim of care from the particular dependent other(s) is 'compelling regardless of universal principles' (Held, 2006, p. 10). From this emphasis on responsibility for the vulnerable and particular other, it is assumed that care ethics advocates partiality. Partiality and care ethics will be subjects for discussion later in this chapter, where some deeper structural problems of care ethics as a normative position will be discussed. These problems relate both to partiality and to the way justice is comprehended in care ethics. It will be shown that even if care ethics to some extent advocates partiality, it fails to accommodate for the particularities of professional caring work. And this analogue problem between the personal and the professional is the main challenge to overcome if care ethics is to be adapted to professional ethics.

The second characteristic of care ethics concerns its underscoring of the moral significance of cultivating emotions, such as sympathy, empathy, sensitivity, and responsiveness, as guidance for morality (Held, 2006). The cultivation of emotions is considered by care ethicists to be important for comprehending a moral situation and also for understanding what is best to do in that situation. Proponents of care ethics characteristically contrast their view with traditional rationalistic moral theories at this point. Held is no exception when she writes:

> The emotions that are typically considered and rejected in rationalist moral theories are the egoistic feelings that undermine universal moral norms, the favouritism that interferes with impartiality, and the aggressive and vengeful impulses for which morality is to provide restraints. The ethics of care, in contrast, typically appreciates the emotions and relational capabilities that enable morally concerned persons in actual interpersonal contexts to understand what would be best.
>
> (Held, 2006, pp. 10–11)

Well aware of possible undesired or misguided emotions, such as self-sacrificing or manipulating others, it is emphasised that there is a need for an *ethics* of care: This point is of course of utmost importance in every caring relationship, whether it is private or professional. As for instance in nursing care, it is assumed that emotions do play an indispensable part in the perception of the patient's subjective needs, especially in the perception of a patient's moral realities such as suffering and pain.[1]

The emphasis on emotions as a significant normative element in care has interesting bearing upon an argument for partiality based on closeness. According to Held (2006), many feminist care ethicists argue that emotions have an important function in developing moral understanding itself, in helping us decide what the recommendations of morality themselves ought to be. According to this perspective, emotions have a normative impact. The point here is that emotional experiences, and subsequently the perception of what is morally at stake, come about in face-to-face situations, in relational and spatio-temporal proximity to the care-receiver, and shape the caring situation. Hence, as Nortvedt emphasises,

> there is an important point here of arguing for economical and organizational conditions of health care that do not violate these basic values of human proximity but show respect for the moral nature of health care as this is tied to individual care in concrete situations.
>
> (Nortvedt, 2012, p. 14)

I come back to proximity-based arguments for partiality in Chapter 5.

An ethics of care calls into question the universalistic, impartial, and abstract rules of dominant systematic moral theories. This is the third characteristic that Held (2006) brings up. The target is what commonly is referred to as an ethics of justice. The moral psychological insights introduced by Gilligan are typically considered as the foundation of care ethics. This is where moral reasoning on care was contrasted with – at that time – dominant moral reasoning based on rights, fairness, and equality. Gilligan used the term 'ethics of justice' to refer to Kohlberg's highest stages of moral development. Hence, an ethics of justice is no single moral theory or a single moral perspective, but includes moral perspectives that focus on equality, fairness, rights, and principles. Care ethicists usually consider the compelling moral claim of the particular other to be morally authoritative even when it conflicts with claims of an ethics of justice. The normative implication of particularity indicated here points to some form and degree of partiality. Other moral philosophers in addition to those traditionally considered as care ethicists have made similar points. Among them are Williams, Blum, and Scheffler,[2] probably the most celebrated theorists on this topic. As already mentioned, an ethics of care has been considered somewhat problematic in a structural normative sense, and I will discuss this issue a bit later. A related problem is that an ethics of care can be somewhat indefinite in its conception of (an ethics of) justice. This will be the topic later in this chapter.

Fourth, an ethics of care calls attention to the moral issues that arise in the private domains of our lives and reconciles the dichotomy of the private and public spheres of morality. This is also a point where care ethicists typically contrast their position with what they refer to as dominant moral theories. Held notes: '[D]ominant theories have assumed that morality should be sought for unrelated, independent, and mutually indifferent individuals assumed to be equal' (Held, 2006, p. 13).

Care ethics, on the other hand, addresses 'moral issues arising in relations among the unequal and dependent, relations that are often emotion-laden and involuntary, and then notices how often these attributes apply not only in the household but in the wider society as well' (Held, 2006, p. 13). However, care ethics fails to accommodate adequately for the role of care within professional relationships. I shall return to this problem in the next section.

The fifth characteristic of an ethics of care concerns its conception of persons and autonomy. Care ethics regards persons as relational and inter-dependent individuals. It denies that persons are self-sufficient and (mutually) independent individuals. Rather, it claims that our social relationships are what make it possible for us to be autonomous and to reason independently and rationally (Held, 2006). Here, again, my claim will be that this position falls short when it comes to comprehending professional roles and dependency in professional relationships.

The overall aim of the next two sections is to discuss whether, and to what extent, care ethics might be able to be adapted for professional ethics. The problems related to the conception of justice and its ambiguity as a normative position according to the care ethics position will be the topic in the next section. In the section 'Mature care, the analogue problem, and moral conflicts', I turn to a discussion of what can be called the analogue problem – that is, to what extent care ethics can be adapted to professional contexts, and by extension to partiality in professional care.

Justice and care: a normative problem of care ethics

The discussions about ethics of care and ethics of justice are numerous and diverse.[3] I do not intend to deal in depth with these debates, but rather to attend to some general points of importance for professional ethics. First I give a brief outline of the discussion's origin. Afterwards I will turn to a discussion on the normativity of care ethics, especially with regard to partiality and professional ethics.

Gilligan was highly critical of the results from studies on moral development conducted by Lawrence Kohlberg, who was her initial supervisor and with whom she worked during the 1970s. Kohlberg's empirical studies on moral reasoning and moral development gave rise to his identification of six stages of moral development. Inspired mainly by Piaget's work on the development of moral judgment, during the mid-1950s Kohlberg conducted several longitudinal studies on moral reasoning from childhood to adulthood (Kohlberg, 1981). By presenting a series of moral dilemmas to his respondents, he discovered a pattern of moral reasoning[4] compatible with a six-stage progression from childhood to adulthood. Gilligan's main critique, which also provided the impetus for her own research, was the emphasis Kohlberg placed on justice as the highest stage of moral development. A related critique from Gilligan was a near-exclusion of women in Kohlberg's sample of respondents:

> Kohlberg's (1958, 1981) six stages that describe the development of moral judgment from childhood to adulthood are based empirically on a study of eighty-four boys whose development Kohlberg has followed for a period of over twenty years. Although Kohlberg claims universality for his stage sequence, those groups not included in his original sample rarely reached his higher stages (Edwards, 1975; Holstein, 1976; Simpson, 1974). Prominent among those who thus appeared to be deficient in moral development when measured by Kohlberg's scale are women, whose judgments seem to exemplify the third stage of his six stage sequence. At this stage morality is conceived in interpersonal terms and goodness is equated with helping and pleasing others.
>
> (Gilligan, 1982, p. 18)

Kohlberg's six stages are grouped into three levels, each of which contains two stages of development. The pre-conventional level represents the two earliest stages of moral development, and is characterised primarily by an egocentric orientation, but there is also, at stage two, a recognition of other people's interests and an awareness of possible conflicting interests (Kohlberg, 1981). Then the progression takes us to the conventional level, consisting of stages three and four. At stage three, moral reasoning is characteristically oriented towards empathy and affection for family members and others (Barry, 1995, p. 236). At stage four, the individual typically takes the point of view of the social system, focusing on roles and duties (Kohlberg, 1981). Finally, there is the post-conventional level, also called the principled level, where 'moral decisions are generated from rights, values, or principles that are (or could be) agreeable to all individuals composing or creating a society designed to have fair and beneficial practices' (Kohlberg, 1981, p. 411). Stages five and six at this level are described as morally superior to the earlier stages. In short, moral reasoning at stage five is marked by equal concern for everyone's interests, and it is a stage of emphasis on the social contract, a perspective that resembles utilitarianism: 'One is concerned that laws and duties be based on rational calculation of overall utility' (Kohlberg, 1981, p. 412). Kantian or Rawlsian ideas of fair treatment of persons feature in the moral reasoning at stage six (Barry, 1995). Kohlberg termed stage six 'the stage of universal ethical principles' (Kohlberg, 1981, p. 412). At this stage, one is a rational person who has seen the validity of universal principles and is committed to them; 'principles are universal principles of justice, the equality of human rights and respect for the dignity of human beings as individuals' (Kohlberg, 1981, p. 412). Kohlberg found that men were much more likely to reason from universal, impartial principles and rules, thereby reaching stages five and six in their moral development. The moral development of women, on the other hand, rarely reached any higher than stage three on his moral development scale of reasoning. Gilligan's own research led to her main claim that stages prior to Kohlberg's stages five and six, especially stage three, represented just as high a level of moral development as did stages five and six. Feminist philosophers found that Gilligan's work resonated with much of their dissatisfaction with dominant moral theories (Held, 2006).

Gilligan argued that Kohlberg's highest level of moral reasoning and judgments represent an ethics of justice that is contrasted to an ethics of care, and that these two moral perspectives are in conflict. Many of Gilligan's feminist successors, along with later critics of impartialist ethics, hold that these perspectives are rival moral outlooks. Others, such as Barry (1995), dispute this claim, arguing that as long as these two approaches to ethical thinking are understood properly, they do not need to be in conflict. We should keep in mind that Gilligan's research consisted of studies in moral psychology, not moral philosophy, and her critique of Kohlberg's work was probably never meant to be very sophisticated philosophically.[5] Additionally, as Held correctly states, '[b]y now, the ethics of care has moved far beyond its original formulations, and any attempt to evaluate it should consider much more than the one or two early works so frequently cited' (Held, 2006, p. 9). Yet, some ambiguities from the earlier period persist.

For instance, care ethics seems to assume two contradictory normative claims:

(a) One normative claim of care ethics is the emphasis on equal concern for the needs and interests of anyone affected by a morally difficult situation (Pettersen, 2008).[6] Held, who otherwise seems to endorse partiality over impartial calculations, says, '[t]he care that is valued by the ethics of care can – and to be justifiable must – include caring for distant others in an interdependent world, and caring that the rights of all are respected and their needs met' (Held, 2006, p. 66). This claim might be illustrative of care ethics' comprehension of justice (not to be confused with an 'ethics of justice'). In that case, care ethics bears some resemblance to a basic form of utilitarianism. But it also might imply a comprehension of justice as fairness, which also requires and aspires to impartiality and universality.[7] In any case, it is not clear what the normative implications here should be.

(b) Another normative claim emphasised in care ethics is 'on the compelling moral salience of attending to and meeting the needs of the particular others for whom we take responsibility' (Held, 2006, p. 10). In earlier writing on feminist[8] care ethics, Held states that '[w]here the conflict is between actual relationship and abstract principle, a feminist approach to morality might give a felt relationship of trust priority over principle and seek morality compatible with this priority' Held, 1995, p. 159). The normative significance care ethicists ascribe to relational care inevitably raises question about partiality (Nortvedt et al., 2011). Care ethics might be taken to imply normative ascription to both impartiality and partiality. There is a rather unclear normative qualification of the link between justice (as impartiality) and relational care (as partiality) both internal to care ethics and between care ethics and ethics of justice.

Interestingly, a strong emphasis on concern for particular, vulnerable others within our 'web of relationships' reflects some form of a principle-based approach to ethics. Kymlicka notes:

> The question, then, is not whether we need principles, but rather what sort of principles. As I noted earlier, some writers have suggested that we face a basic choice between principles of 'rights and fairness' (in the justice approach), or principles of 'responsibilities and relationships' (in the care perspective).
>
> (Kymlicka, 2002, p. 404)

This might appear to be a paradox. But, of course, one could say that care ethics *in principle* emphasises responsibility and relationships without thereby being a *principle-based* ethical outlook. At the same time, care ethicists cannot ignore the importance of 'rights and fairness' even within a non-principle-based perspective. Although Gilligan and other care ethicists emphasise that the care perspective is about responsibilities rather than rights, it seems quite odd to say that an ethics of care is not interested in the rights of other people. A concern for the care receiver's (and the caregiver's) rights must be an integral part of caring. But the point of issue in care ethics is that responsibility for the vulnerable other goes beyond rational accounts of moral obligations and moral or other kinds of rights. In other words, concerns for rights and fairness are *in principle* not the front line for proponents of care ethics. Here a difficulty concerning the scope of care ethics becomes evident. Caring in private and personal relationships is not based on the notion of rights protection, concerns about fairness, equality, etc. A father caring for his child does not, I presume, do so primarily because he as a father has a moral and legal duty to take care of his child's rights to adequate nutrition and hygiene, mental stimulation, protection from harm, etc. Caring in personal and private relationships arises from moral and relational concerns far beyond what can be captured in verbal or written language, and certainly far beyond what can be captured in the technical language of rights and duties.

But in professional care this sense of concern is somewhat different. Perhaps this is why care ethics struggles to accommodate to contexts of professional care. First, professional relationships are structured role relationships where the professional roles are defined prior to the establishment of the relationship.

That is, the existence of a professional relationship is dependent on the pre-definition and establishment of the relevant roles in question, for instance a nurse and a patient. A patient does not, at least ordinarily, seek professional health-care workers for reasons other than their medical needs (Nordhaug and Nortvedt, 2011a). Without the patient's particular needs for medical treatment and/or nursing care, and the professional's expert knowledge and obligations to pursue the 'collective goods' of the profession, the professional relationship would not exist. This is also why the professional relationship is asymmetrical in a different sense to many caring relationships in the private domain. The asymmetry in knowledge and competency between the nurse and patient reflects a critical asymmetry in power and vulnerability (Nordhaug and Nortvedt, 2011b). Professional obligations to patients are also, of course, restricted by ethical guidelines that emphasise impartiality and equality. In professional care, as contrasted to personal care, moral responsibilities are framed by the distinctive areas of professional concerns, such as medical needs or the need for nursing care. Hence, if the scope of care ethics is to include professional care, it has to incorporate the more principle-based perspectives underlying such care work. As Held notes, 'partiality and the value of caring relation-ships are not the only values of concern to morality. The social conventions through which partiality is practiced need to be evaluated and justified, and impartial moral principles can be relevant in doing so' (Held, 2006, p. 96). Later in this chapter I suggest that ethics of nursing care should endorse a prerogative for partiality, and then in Chapter 6 I turn to a discussion of how such a prerogative could be balanced with claims of impartial concerns such as fairness.

Nursing, Nelson argues, requires 'an ethics that is sensitive to the particulars of a given personal relationship yet still leaves room for action in the wider society. It requires, in short, a *particularistic* rather than a *partialist* ethics' (Nelson, 1992, p. 12). While some writers on care ethics, such as Bubeck (1995) find the association between care ethics and particularism unfortunate, care ethics seems to be a moderate particularistic[9] ethical outlook, but advocat-ing a certain prerogative for partial concerns. Still, care ethics appears internally inconsistent, and its proponents need to clarify what follows from its basic theoretical assumptions about the normative role of partiality in ethics, espe-cially as regards professional ethics. The relational interdependency empha-sised in care ethics can also be related to the notion of reciprocity found in the concept of mature care. Mature care is a virtue-based *normative* concept recently introduced in care ethics. The next section addresses these issues.

Mature care, the analogue problem, and moral conflicts

One recent and important contribution to the normative discussions of care ethics stems from Pettersen (2008). The concept of mature care originates from Gilligan's work on moral psychological development. But the normative implications of the concept were first developed by Tove Pettersen two decades later. By exploring and developing the concept of mature care, Pettersen has also contributed to a substantial development of care ethics. In treating care as a virtue, the essence of mature care is an emphasis on reciprocity where the mature agent has the ability to balance concerns for oneself with those of others and act from a principle of not harming (Pettersen, 2008; Pettersen and Hem, 2011; Nordhaug and Nortvedt, 2011b).

An article by Nortvedt and myself (2011b) explores and discusses some challenges of applying the concept of mature care into contexts of nursing care and health care prioritisations. I will base the discussion in this chapter on the two main problems identified in this article. The first problem is what I take to be an overemphasis on reciprocity in caring relationships. The second challenge relates to situations of moral conflict and difficult moral choices.

In relation to professional ethics, mature care is so far primarily discussed as an alternative to prevailing altruistic concepts of care. Reciprocity, as the importance of balancing the needs and interests of the caregiver against those of the care receiver, is the main issue in these discussions.[10] Based on the concern that an overemphasis on altruism generates self-sacrifice and selflessness on behalf of the caregiver, mature care is introduced as an alternative to altruistic concepts of care. Pettersen writes:

> Intuitively we tend to understand 'care' as care for others, and that the more other-directed care is, the better. The notion of mature care, how-ever, involves as much concern for oneself as it does for others. Mature care implies a balancing between the interests of self and others.
>
> (Pettersen, 2008, p. 14)

We should note that Pettersen does not object to the importance of an altruistic component in professional care work. Her critique seems to be that altruistic approaches to care are too vague and unreliable as regards motiva-tion. As she correctly observes, true altruistic callings may motivate some care workers, but there is also a wide range of other motives, such as vocation and self-realisation, and instrumental reasons. The problem then is to distinguish between these different motivations for caring and then determine whether or not the caregiver is motivated by altruism (Pettersen, 2008). But as Bubeck points out, it is difficult to imagine anybody choosing a caring profession unless they had some sort of personal commitment, at least initially, to a vocation that involved caring. Besides, he notes:

> one of the main differences between public and private care is that public care fails to meet the conditions which would allow for fully individua-lized, 'particular' care: it is not motivated by existing particular relation-ships and an impulse to act on behalf of the other on the basis of this relationship and the emotions appropriate to it, nor can it use the indivi-dualized knowledge that persons who know each other typically have of each other. It is nevertheless a response to needs, informed by general

knowledge and motivated by a general commitment to care for those in need.

(Bubeck, 1995, p. 219)

Additionally, the assertion is that altruistic care may lead to self-sacrifice and selflessness. This is why mature care is the suggested alternative. Pettersen says:

As a virtue, mature care is not the opposite of vice; it is not the other side of selfish or selfless acts or emotions. Mature care is characterized by its intermediate position, it is the mean between too little and too much concern for others (or for oneself). In care-work, selfishness is likely to correlate with indifference to and ignorance of the patients in one's care. It can result in harm. Self-sacrifice, at the other extreme, (apparently caring too much for others) encourages a paternalistic approach, and increases the danger of violating the patient's autonomy.

(Pettersen, 2008, p. 125)

Although I agree with the main points offered here, I think there is an over-emphasis on reciprocity, which causes problems when the concept of mature care is applied to a professional health care context. Professional care work is principally other-directed and is concerned about balancing other–other concerns, not self–other concerns. This is not to say that health care professionals should ignore their own interests and needs, but limits should not be set in a way that compromises the legitimate needs of patients (Nordhaug and Nortvedt, 2011b). I will keep to the claim that this critique is founded on an overly absolute interpretation of altruistic care, at least in the context of professional care.

As part of this reply, I would advocate Blum's definition of altruism as a more suitable description of the form of altruism that characterises nursing care. In Blum's words, '[b]y "altruism" I will mean a regard for the good of another person for his own sake, or conduct motivated by such regard' (Blum, 1980, pp. 9–10). However, as stated earlier, this definition departs from the customary use of the concept in that a connotation of self-sacrifice or self-neglect is not a part of it. Perhaps this is more important in professional care work, which is basically asymmetrical in power and vulnerability, as mentioned earlier, compared to personal relationships. Professional care work, such as nursing, could be described in terms of generalised reciprocity.[11] Generalised reciprocity entails showing concern, attention, and care for another, for the other's sake, without expecting anything in return. The professional duties and responsibilities undertaken by a nurse also entail that he or she cannot (and should not) expect anything in return from the patient. But it does not follow from this that the nurse sacrifices or neglects her or himself, or anything of value to her or him. Hence, generalised reciprocity resembles Blum's definition of altruism.

As mentioned above, a problem here is that care ethics has failed to accommodate the particularities characterising a professional relationship such as between a nurse and a patient. A professional relationship is in several important senses of a different nature than the attachments and loyalties within personal relationships. A relationship between a nurse and a patient is a structured relationship where the roles as well as the direction of care are defined and fixed prior to the establishment of the relationship (Nordhaug and Nortvedt, 2011a). This is not necessarily the case in personal relationships. Consider two archetypical personal relationships: parenthood and friendship. In parenthood, the roles and the direction of care are defined prior to the establishment of the relationship between parent and child. But neither the roles nor the direction of care are fixed. In fact they may very well change during a lifespan as the parent and the child grow older. In friendship, the roles and the direction of care are also dynamic. While personal relationships may differ to some extent, they share the characteristic of being intrinsically (morally) valuable to us. Personal relationships are sources of vulnerability and dependency; they can fail, and they can be oppressive (Nortvedt et al., 2011), but they are also genuinely valuable. As part of Scheffler's normative position, such a non-instrumental value of personal relationships will be discussed in the next chapter. The moral value of a professional relationship is first and foremost based on the good provided by the professional. Care in personal relationships is grounded in existing relatedness, but in professional relationships care is not (and should not) be grounded in *existing* (personal) relatedness. The professional relationship is focussed on a particular good that both parties wish – or usually wish – to promote (Koehn, 1994).

Against this background, the problem with care ethics in professional contexts arises. The human interdependency emphasised by care ethics is significantly different in professional relationships. This is not to deny that nurses as well as patients indeed are interdependent as human beings. But within the context of a professional relationship, the interdependency is restricted to the roles in question, to the particular caring situation, as well as to how the relationship evolves in space and time. As already noted, the role of a nurse and the role of a patient are both somehow *replaceable*. While personal aspects of care, such as a certain kind of emotional bonding, might be a significant part of a professional relationship (especially in long-term care, rehabilitation units, etc.), this is not generally what *constitutes* it. What constitutes a relationship between a nurse and a patient is the patient's need for nursing care, and the nurse's ability to meet these needs.

The importance of balancing the needs and interests of the caregiver against those of the care receiver is one of the main issues in mature care. This also represents the most prominent issue when adapting mature care to professional ethics (Nordhaug and Nortvedt, 2011b). This balancing seems to imply that the interests and needs of both caregiver and care receiver are of equal importance and moral value. This is of course not a genuine problem in itself. It is perfectly in line with general ideas about equality. The problem arises because mature care does not address how these needs and interests should be weighed and counterbalanced (Nordhaug and Nortvedt, 2011b).

According to Pettersen, the balancing requires 'a judgment that implies contextual sensitivity and consideration of the needs of the recipient and that of the care giver' (Pettersen, 2008, p. 146).

And here the second problem of mature care in professional contexts becomes apparent. The main problem of mature care as a normative outlook in professional care is that the concept is less useful in situations where it is difficult or even impossible to *harmonise* the interests and needs of different patients (Nordhaug and Nortvedt, 2011b). In nursing care, the main challenge is not to balance the needs and interests of oneself as a nurse with the needs of the patient. The predicament is rather to balance different concerns for patients: 'To argue for the distinction between health care professionals' interests versus those of patients as the dominant consideration would be to misconstrue what professional health care is about, namely caring for sick patients, not for professionals' (Nordhaug and Nortvedt, 2011b, p. 210). Hence, reciprocity is a problematical normative ideal in nursing care.

I will not argue for the neglect of professionals' needs and interests in a caring situation. Instead, the interests and needs of the professional should mainly be viewed as those interests and needs one has *as a professional* (Nordhaug and Nortvedt, 2011b). It seems reasonable to say that, very often, and mainly, the interest one has *as a professional* in a caring situation is in line with the patient's interest in that very same situation. For instance, both the nurse and the patient may have a joint goal of getting the patient's wound healed, or that the patient is able to walk from the bed to the bathroom with some assistance, to mention a couple of nursing projects. Then, there is no conflict between the interests of the nurse and the patient; however, these interests may conflict with the interests of other patients (Nordhaug and Nortvedt, 2011b). And this conflict, which frequently arises due to resource constraints, could cause professional self-sacrifice because: 'professionals are not able to perform their tasks and discharge their responsibilities to their patients. The main problem, then, is not altruistic care, but lack of resources to provide proper nursing care' (Nordhaug and Nortvedt, 2011b, p. 213).

Perhaps, then, we could say that a very important insight of mature care could be that nurses should balance their interests and needs not so much with those of the patients, but with economic and organisational concerns and interests.

The question of how to reconcile divergent interests and needs is yet unanswered. Although prevention of conflicts, rather than conflict solving, is the focus in care ethics (Pettersen, 2008), the position has to come to grips with the question of how one balances multiple needs.

> On one level we can think of human neediness as a part of the tragedy of human existence: there will inevitably be more care needs than can be met. In meeting some needs, other needs will inevitably go unmet. Since caring rests upon the satisfaction of needs for care, the problem of determining which needs should be met shows that the care ethic is not individualistic,

but must be situated in the broader moral context. Obviously a theory of justice is necessary to discern among more or less urgent needs. Yet the kind of theory of justice that will be necessary to determine needs is probably different from most current theories of justice. Some of the most difficult questions within the moral framework of care arise out of trying to determine what 'needs' should mean and how competing needs should be evaluated and met.

(Tronto, 1993, pp. 137–138)

When confronted with a moral dilemma, mature agents are able to balance all the needs and interests involved. The agent's aim is to avoid harming oneself and others, and to promote well-being (Pettersen, 2008). To be able to do this, mature agents make decisions and act according to contextual sensitivity and idiosyncratic information acquired through communication and dialogue (Pettersen, 2008, p. 91). While I am sympathetic to this account of moral conflict and dilemmas, a crucial question of normativity remains, both for mature care and for care ethics in general: Due to the ambitiously defined web of relationships that constitute our moral responsibilities, how are we to decide who is involved and who is vulnerable in a particular situation? Besides, if mature care involves informing agents in difficult situations, it must address and justify what are the most relevant concerns for moral judgments in particular contexts and situations. It seems, however, unclear in what way mature care can address conflicts such as those outlined above without accepting more principle-based procedures for priority decisions grounded in other ethical concepts such as deontology or consequentialism (Nordhaug and Nortvedt, 2011b). This is not only a challenge for mature care; perhaps it is even a greater problem for care ethics in general due to its ambiguous normative perspectives.

A normative shift towards a more principle-based care ethics is needed for its prospects as a plausible ethical outlook in nursing care. In the final chapter of this book I explore and attempt to outline an ethical outlook for nursing care that incorporates particularistic and principle-based moral perspectives. According to Bubeck, there are in particular two principles that caregivers in the public sphere follow. The one most obvious, according to Bubeck, is a principle of harm minimisation.[12] Chapter 5 deals with deontological constraints on what a nurse is permitted to do. Here, a principle of not harming can also serve as an argument for partiality. And then as a prolongation of that argument I turn to a discussion of consequentialism by the end of that chapter. The second principle Bubeck suggests for care ethics is the principle of equality – a principle, he says, which is not always compatible with that of harm minimisation. In Chapter 6 I discuss a principle of equality that is a fundamental principle for distributing health care resources. My aim is to establish an argument stating that partiality does not have to be inconsistent with either a principle of equality or a principle of harm minimisation as long as partiality is permissible.

Conclusion on care ethics in professional care

So far in this chapter I have discussed two main challenges that arise when applying care ethics in the context of professional care. My argument was motivated by the strong focus on the part of care ethics on relational care and responsibility. What we have here is a moral perspective stating the significance not of consequences, rules, and duties, or (with some exceptions) virtues, but of how relationships generate responsibility to care for the vulnerable other. For this reason I first assumed that care ethics advocates for partiality. I remain agnostic to whether it really does, particularly because the literature on care ethics presents an indistinct normative position. Care ethics has a rather confusing account of justice. It highlights the importance of equal concern for all involved, and our moral responsibility to anyone within our web of relationships. The normative significance of our relational web is, however, undefined. In some important way care ethics can be taken to argue for a quite narrow web that includes only the more personal face-to-face relationships. At the same time, it seems to be a moderate particularistic moral perspective. It does not shut the doors on impartial and universal considerations of justice in moral reasoning, but stresses the importance of contextual information combined with a concern for anyone affected. Still, care ethics seems to *in principle* be against the idea that principle-based moral perspectives matter the most for moral judgments. The questions, then, to which there are no adequate answers, are which concerns matter the most and why. And here the second challenge discussed becomes evident. Care ethics has a hard time accommodating the particular features that characterise professional relationships. If the scope of care also entails care for those with particular, professional needs, care ethics should be adjusted for a more principle-based account. As Bubeck also points out, principles of justice in care take on a more prominent role in care in the public sphere (Bubeck, 1995). For instance, as a nurse I have responsibility for any patient with a legitimate need for nursing care. I am all these patients' keeper. At the same time, I cannot care for all patients at the same time. Care ethics emphasises contextual information as a fundamental source of decision-making. But what should I emphasise? How should I balance divergent concerns? What matters more or less, and who is affected: only the patient in front of me, or other patients, relatives, colleagues, or perhaps the organisation or economic sustainability?

In the next chapter I aim to advance an argument for partiality based on proximity. And then, in Chapter 6, I discuss how such an argument can and should be balanced against concerns for justice.

Notes

1 For an important contribution on the topic of moral realism in clinical health care, see Nortvedt (2012).
2 See Williams (1985/1993); Blum (1980); Scheffler (2001) and (2010).

3 There are also many approaches to a typology of the differences between ethics of care and ethics of justice. Some contributions are Kymlicka (2002) and Dancy (1992)
4 Neither Kohlberg nor Gilligan was particularly focussed on their respondents' *conclusions* per se when making moral judgments. For both of them, the emphasis was on moral reasoning, and the link between moral reasoning and moral judgment.
5 See for instance Pettersen (2008).
6 This is also what lies behind the arising of moral dilemmas. According to Pettersen 'what characterizes a moral dilemma within the morality of care is how to care for everybody at the same time'(Pettersen, 2008, p. 91).
7 Perhaps there are some similarities also between care ethics and other moral positions in which universality and impartiality are central. See for instance Kymlicka (2002, p. 408) for a comparison of care ethics and the requirements of Rawls's account of the original position.
8 Care ethicists need not adhere to feminism to accept this claim.
9 Moderate particularism is here taken to denote Blum's pluralistic account of particularism: 'The philosophical account thus provides for recognizing multiple moral concerns, including those of a non-particularist and non-partialist nature. It therefore bids a moral agent reflect on her aims and dispositions. It does not promote the conception of particularity as mindlessly following one's emotions and inclinations and intuitions of the moment. At the same time it recognizes, as none of the impartialist projects discussed here do, that various sort of particularistic and partialist motives, sentiments, and perceptions are source of moral or ethical value distinct from that provided by impartialist theories, and are no more fundamental to the moral life and to theories thereof' (Blum, 2000, p. 226).
10 See for instance Pettersen (2008); Hem (2008); and Pettersen and Hem (2011).
11 See for instance pp. 71–75 in Martinsen (1989).
12 According to Bubeck (1995) this is also, under circumstances of justice, a principle of distributive justice since it allows for a decision on whose needs should be given preference.

References

Andolsen, B., 2001. Care and justice as moral values for nurses in an era of managed care. In: Cates, D. and Lauritzen, P., eds, *Medicine and the ethics of care*. Washington, DC: Georgetown University Press, pp. 41–68.
Barry, B., 1995. *A treatise on social justce. Volume II. Justice as impartiality*. Oxford: Clarendon Press.
Blum, L., 1980. *Friendship, altruism and morality*. London: Routledge & Kegan Paul.
Blum, L., 2000. Against deriving particularity. In: Hooker, B. and Little, M., eds, *Moral particularism*. New York: Oxford University Press, pp. 205–226.
Bubeck, D., 1995. *Care, gender, and justice*. Oxford: Clarendon Press.
Dancy, J., 1992. Caring about justice. *Philosophy*, 67(262), pp. 447–466.
Darwall, S., 1998. *Philosophical ethics*. Boulder, CO: Westview Press.
Gilligan, C., 1982. *In a different voice: Psychological theory and women's development*. London: Harvard University Press.
Held, V., 1995. Feminist moral inquiry and the feminist future [1993]. In: Held, V., ed., *Justice and care: Essential reading in feminist ethics*. Boulder, CO: Westview Press, pp. 153–176.
Held, V., 2006. *The ethics of care: Personal, political, and global*. Oxford: Oxford University Press.

Hem, M., 2008. Mature care? An empirical study of interaction between psychotic patients and psychiatric nurses. Dissertaion, University of Oslo.

Koehn, D., 1994. *The ground of professional ethics.* London: Routledge

Kohlberg, L., 1981. *The philosophy of moral development.* Cambridge: Harper & Row.

Korsgaard, C., 1996. The normative question. In: Korsgaard, C., ed., *The sources of normativity.* Cambridge: Cambridge University Press, pp. 7–48.

Kymlicka, W., 2002. *Contemporary political philosophy.* 2nd edn. New York: Oxford University Press.

Martinsen, K., 1989. *Omsorg, sykepleie og medisin: Historisk-filosofiske essays.* Oslo: Tano [Norwegian].

Nelson, H., 1992. Against caring. *The Journal of Clinical Etihcs,* 3(1), pp. 8–20.

Nordhaug, M. and Nortvedt, P., 2011a. Justice and proximity: Problems for an ethics of care. *Health Care Analysis,* 19, pp. 3–14.

Nordhaug, M. and Nortvedt, P., 2011b. Mature care in professional relationships and health care prioritizations. *Nursing Ethics,* 18(2), pp. 209–216.

Nortvedt, P., 2012. The normativity of clinical health care: Perspectives on moral realism. *Journal of Medicine and Philosophy,* 37(3), pp. 295–309.

Nortvedt, P., Hem, M. and Skirbekk, H., 2011. The ethics of care: Role obligations and moderate partiality in health care. *Nursing Ethics,* 18(2), pp. 192–200.

Pettersen, T., 2008. *Comprehending care: Problems and possibilities in the ethics of care.* Lanham, MD: Lexington Books.

Pettersen, T. and Hem, M., 2011. Mature care and reciprocity: Two cases from acute psychiatry. *Nursing Ethics,* 18(2), pp. 217–231.

Rawls, J., 1971. *A theory of justice.* s. l. Cambridge, MA: Harvard University Press.

Scheffler, S., 2001. *Boundaries and allegiances.* Oxford: Oxford University Press.

Scheffler, S., 2010. *Equality and tradition.* New York: Oxford University Press.

Tronto, J., 1993. *Moral boundaries: A political argument for an ethic of care.* New York: Routledge.

Williams, B., 1985/1993. *Ethics and the limits of philosophy.* London: Routledge.

5 Towards a prerogative for partiality in nursing care

By a critique of consequentialism Scheffler (2001; 2010) explores the normative significance of those things in life that we value and that are valuable to us. In particular he investigates the normative implications of our personal relationships and our personal projects. The most important implication is that our relationships and – to some extent – our projects give rise to special duties (partiality) that cannot always be trumped by impartial concerns of consequentialism. Scheffler does not discuss whether his arguments are applicable to professional relationships and professional projects. And since Scheffler's account is premised on what agents as persons value and what agents have reason to value, the analogue between personal relationships and professional relationships is the main challenge to accept here. It would be radical and controversial to claim and presuppose that nurses in fact *personally* value their relationships with their patients, as a friend values his relationship to his friend. My claim here will be that nurses *as nurses* have reason to value the nursing project. Note that this argument does not presuppose that nurses in fact do so. It is a normative statement, not an empirical one. The nursing project can only be fulfilled in the concrete encounter and relationship between a nurse and her patient. Such a project of professional care is also valuable from an objective point of view since it is the fundament upon which the nursing profession as part of institutional health care is built. Individualised and relational nursing care is valuable, and morally desirable, or so I shall argue. In fact, some notions of partialist concerns for patients might be essential if nurses are to discharge their professional commitment of individualised and adequate nursing care.

The normative value of what we care about

> As a matter of fact, the observation that there is an element of 'forbidden fruit' in love and friendship, according to consequentialism, is as it should be. This is something most people testify that they feel when, in a world of starvation, they watch TV and show special concern for their near and dear.
>
> (Tännsjö, 1995, p. 127)

Previously, I discussed role-relative reasons for partiality. It was shown that partiality in nursing-care might be based on role-relative reasons that either could be formulated in general terms (reasons that apply to any nurse) or as reasons that apply to a nurse, but not necessarily any nurse, in a particular situation. In this section, I consider arguments alluding to some sort of role-relativity and partiality in nursing care. The main challenge is how such arguments fit into professional ethics. I will begin with Scheffler's arguments for the normative significance of relationships.

Scheffler explores the normative significance of interpersonal relationships from the perspective of what he calls common-sense moral thought or common-sense moralities. His main argument is that the non-instrumental valuing of personal relationships generates special responsibilities[1] to those with whom we share these particular relationships. Scheffler describes non-instrumental valuing along these lines:

> if I have a special, valued relationship with someone, and if the value I attach to the relationship is not purely instrumental in character – if, in other words, I do not value it solely as a means to some independently specified end – then I regard the person with whom I have the relationship as capable of making additional claims on me, beyond those that people in general can make. For to attach non-instrumental value to my relationship with a particular person just is, in part, to see that person as a source of special claims in virtue of the relationship between us. It is, in other words, to be disposed, in contexts which vary depending on the nature of the relationship, to see that person's needs, interests, and desires as, in themselves, providing me with presumptively decisive reasons for action, reasons that I would not have had in the absence of the relationship.
>
> (Scheffler, 2001, p. 100)

A central claim is that these relationships could not play the role they do in our lives if they did not also generate special responsibilities (Scheffler, 2001).

According to Scheffler, special responsibilities are additional and sometimes greater responsibilities than general responsibilities towards others. Hence, they cannot fully be reduced to distributive concerns (Scheffler, 2001). Note that this does not mean that special responsibilities necessarily undermine distributive concerns, such as taking the interests of all relevant parties into account (Scheffler, 2001; Nortvedt and Nordhaug, 2008). Special responsibilities are *additional*, i.e. they rather increase our total responsibilities (Scheffler, 2001). But there is something peculiar about this claim. That is, if some responsibilities are stronger than general responsibilities, how then can they be additional? If they are stronger, they trump other concerns. If they are additional, they do not necessarily trump other concerns. A response to this objection is to say that as long as one takes the interests of all relevant parties into account, one is permitted to act on the reasons generated by the non-instrumental valuing of a close relationship. Hence, the responsibilities generated from the non-instrumental valuing are only additional to, but not necessarily stronger than, our general responsibilities. To say that special responsibilities are additional seems to me only to make sense when there is no conflict of interest or when one's resources in some way are too scarce to fulfil both one's special responsibilities and one's general responsibilities. Nevertheless, I think it suffices for the discussion to say that special responsibilities are to some extent *stronger* than general responsibilities.

Special responsibilities are generated from relational attachments. But according to Scheffler there are many different kinds of relationships that might give rise to special responsibilities. Even though they share no obvious feature (e.g. voluntary participation or not), the common feature that gives rise to special responsibility is that these relationships are valued non-instrumentally. For the most part, Scheffler's discussions concern our private lives and personal relationships, but he makes no clear distinction between personal and public groups and relationships. Since it is my purpose to determine whether Scheffler's position is applicable to the debate about partiality in professional contexts, the primary and decisive question is whether professional relationships in particular can be valued non-instrumentally. As I have said previously, the existence (as well as the maintenance) of a professional relationship is based on the patients' medical- and nursing-care needs. Subsequently, there is an important sense in which the relationship between a nurse and a patient is fundamentally instrumental. Consider an example given by Nordhaug and Nortvedt (2011). Tom is a nurse who works in short-staffed nursing home ward. This morning two of the short-term patients were to be discharged to make the rooms ready for new patients. Due to the situational constraints, Tom is unable to provide adequate care for the patients for whom he is responsible:

> One of these patients, Mary, was very anxious about leaving since she lived alone and her family was away on a holiday trip. Tom's professional assessment was that Mary's physical state and self-care could improve greatly if she only could have stayed one more week.
>
> (Nordhaug and Nortvedt, 2011, p. 4)

At the same time, if Mary's stay is extended, the patient waiting for admission to the room would suffer (Nordhaug and Nortvedt, 2011). The question here is, not surprisingly, what should Tom do?

The relationship between Tom and Mary is based on Mary's particular nursing care needs. Without these needs, there would be no relationship between them (there might of course have been a private relationship between them if they had known each other prior to the hospitalisation. But let us assume that this is not the case). The relationship is established because Tom is in a position to help Mary with her particular needs. In actual fact, the relationship between Mary and Tom is established to serve some specified end (representing one or more of the collective goods provided by nursing care).

In this way, the relationship has an instrumental value. From Scheffler's account, then, this relationship gives Tom no *special* responsibility for Mary. In other words, he has no reason – from Scheffler's account – to be partial.

We should bear in mind that Scheffler's argument concerns the valuing of relationships, not the valuing of persons per se. Suppose then, that Tom values his relationship to Mary non-instrumentally.[2] For instance, Mary has been in the ward for quite a long time and Tom has grown to like her as a person; so to him the relationship has an intrinsic and personal value, and he wants to sustain it. Then, from Scheffler's account, Tom has reason to act partially towards her (because this valuing gives rise to special responsibilities that are stronger and greater than his responsibilities to others). Hence, if Tom values the relationship with Mary non-instrumentally, (it must be true that) Tom sees Mary as a source of special claims in virtue of the relationship between himself and Mary. Additionally, Tom must attach value to the relationship, a value that is not purely instrumental in character. Stated differently, to be valued non-instrumentally, the relationship has to acquire something more than instrumental purpose. Here, one can ask: wouldn't this relationship exist independently of the nurse (or the patient) valuing it in one way or another? That is, a professional relationship arises and exists whether or not the caregiver and the care receiver actually *value* the relationship per se. Hence, the requirement of non-instrumental valuing is a real challenge for a proper defence of relational partiality in nursing. First, one might suspect Tom of being partial because of his personal preferences. In that case, he is biased since he values something in his relationship with Mary that he doesn't value in his relationships with other patients. Even more importantly, the opposite must then be true: If Tom does *not* value a relationship with Mary, he has no reason to be partial towards her (according to Scheffler's account). Therefore, if a professional values a relationship with a patient non-instrumentally, we have three possible scenarios:

a   Illegitimate partiality: that is, partiality understood as prejudice or bias (see Chapter 1).
b   Arbitrary partiality: If the relationship in fact is valued non-instrumentally, partiality might be legitimate. The consequence is that partiality might be distributed arbitrarily, i.e. partiality depends upon whether or not the person/nurse values it. With regard to professional ethics, I find this implication unacceptable.
c   Legitimate partiality (provided the relationship in fact is valued non-instrumentally).

Special responsibilities are stronger and go beyond our duties to other people. According to Scheffler, the 'greater strength' of these responsibilities has implications for both our positive duties and our negative duties to other people. Let me mention two such implications. First, 'the positive duties to one's associate often take precedence over one's positive duties to others in cases where the two conflict' (Scheffler, 2001, p. 51). I may sometimes be required to help my brother even if his need is less urgent than the stranger's. In professional care this would imply, for instance, that Tom's co-worker can claim the right to partiality, and prioritise her patient's morning toileting, instead of assisting Tom with the morning toileting of his patient (provided performing the morning toileting of a patient is considered a positive professional duty). Then her right (and her patient's right) to partiality cannot be overruled by the needs of Tom's patient (and Tom's need for assistance). But it would also mean that the positive duties one has to one's own patient can take precedence over the positive duties one has to other, distant patients. Second, 'the threshold at which a positive duty can override a negative duty is sometimes lower if the positive duty is to an associate, than it would be if the positive duty were to a stranger' (Scheffler, 2001, p. 51). This could mean, for instance, that Tom's co-worker can claim the right to partiality, and prioritise her patient's morning toileting, instead of assisting Tom even if his patient's situation should suddenly turn critical. Then her right (and her patient's right) to partiality overrules the needs of Tom's patient (and his need for assistance). Of course, this is problematic since it could imply that some patients' needs are not attended to at all. It is therefore of vital importance that *need-assessment* is part of the professional's reasoning.

Now, in his later writings, Scheffler's (2010) claim is that morality in general incorporates project-dependent, relationship-dependent, and membership-dependent reasons, and thereby accommodates reasonable partiality. According to Scheffler's position, then, valuing a project and a relationship (non-instrumentally) is to see them as sources of reasons for action: 'Personal projects and relationships by their nature define forms of reasonable partiality, partiality not merely in our preferences or affections but in the reasons that flow from some of our most basic values' (Scheffler, 2010, p. 49).

Scheffler argues that both relationships and projects can generate reasons for partiality, but we are only obligated to act on the former (Scheffler, 2010). The two sets of reasons (relationships and projects) are reasons for action, and reasons to form normative expectations of each other. This notion of mutual normativity does not exist in projects, because relationships often entail an entitlement to complain if needs are neglected (Scheffler, 2010). For example:

> If I fail to act on compelling relationship-dependent reasons to attend to my son's needs, then, other things equal, I have wronged him and he has a legitimate complaint against me. But if I fail to act on compelling project-dependent reasons to finish my novel, I have wronged no one and no one is in a privileged position to complain.
>
> (Scheffler, 2010, pp. 52–53)

There can be legitimate reasons to prioritise a project, but that does not mean that anyone will complain if then project is not fulfilled. I think Scheffler might be correct in this claim, but only to the extent that it concerns our private lives. In a professional context, people certainly have reason to complain if a project is not fulfilled; for example, the requirement to fulfil a nursing project, as I mentioned earlier, is a basic obligation of nurses. A patient is definitively part of such a project, and thereby entitled to complain if the project is neglected.

We should bear in mind that Scheffler does not base his arguments on an account of goodness or 'value' as a noun. Scheffler is only concerned with *valuing*. To Scheffler, valuing a project is to see it as justifiable:

> to value a project of one's own is, among other things, to see it as giving one reasons for action in a way that other people's projects do not, and in a way that other comparably valuable activities in which one might engage in do not.
>
> (Scheffler, 2010, p. 48)

This does not mean that one should consider one's own project as more valuable than that of others. Nor does it mean that one's project-dependent reasons always take priority over other reasons:

> Still, if I value my projects non-instrumentally, then I shall see them as a distinctive source of reasons for action, and there will be contexts which I see myself as having reasons to pursue those projects even though doing so means passing up opportunities to engage in other equally valuable activities or to assist other people with their equally valuable projects.
>
> (Scheffler, 2010, p. 48)

Surely the nursing project (see Chapter 2) is morally valuable to the extent that it assures a desirable collective good (either on a public level or an individual level). But I am not sure an argument for a non-instrumental valuing of the project can be established. That is, while nursing care in itself might have a non-instrumental value, for instance, in long-term care where nurses and patients might get to know each other in a more personal sense, in general, nursing care has instrumental value. Indeed, the relationship between a nurse and a patient would not even exist if it was not for instrumental reasons. Hence, a project-based account of professional partiality seems to fail for the same reasons that it proved too complex to justify a normative significance of professional relationships based on Scheffler's premises. The main impediment is the premise of non-instrumental valuing. Still, I will not completely dismiss project-based reasons for partiality. In the next chapter my aim is to advance such an account.

A prerogative of partiality in nursing

In the previous chapter I argued that a relationship-based approach to partiality cannot adequately account for partiality in professional contexts.

Nurse–patient relationships are one of the most central parts of professional health care work, and might in some situations even display a therapeutic value. But it proved difficult to accommodate care ethics to the particularities of these kinds of relationships. The difficulty of care ethics was primarily its ambiguous accounts of normativity and of ethics of justice traditions. Scheffler's position is a more promising normative account for my purpose here, but it was unsuccessfully applied because of its premises. The main problem with Scheffler's relational account here is the premise of non-instrumental valuing of relationships. To be motivated to care for a particular patient for this particular patient's sake does not presuppose a non-instrumental valuing. Although valuing a relationship and the emotional attachments that may arise in nurse–patient relationships certainly can explain partial acts, they do not justify them normatively.

In this section, I presume that professions serve desirable collective goods that members of a community have a joint right to (Miller, 2010, p. 179). In Chapter 2 I said that the collective goods of nursing are represented by the four basic responsibilities of this profession (i.e. to promote health, to prevent illness, to restore health, and to alleviate suffering), and furthermore, that nursing care encapsulates a specific form of caring which is initially focused on the particular caring needs of the patient. At the same time, and based on Blum's account of vocational caring, we could say that nursing care must involve some regard for the overall good of the patient, and a sense of how the good of the nursing activities complies with the patient's overall good (Blum, 1994). From this, we might say that adequate and individualised nursing care for patients is of vital importance if a nurse is to realise the aims of the nursing profession. Based on these presumptions, I now aim to explore and develop an argument for a prerogative for partiality in nursing care.

Later in this chapter we shall see that Scheffler (2010) has made an argument advocating the normative significance of valuable projects. My assumption is that this account is more promising in the context of professional care, but then it cannot be premised on non-instrumental valuing. Normative (action-guiding) professional ethics must obviously have a reference to the orientation and guiding concerns of the profession in question (Oakley and Cocking, 2001). To be action-guiding, professional ethics must then account for the aims of the profession. But the (explanatory) statement above is quite simplified in that it only says that partiality might be a precondition to serve the ends of nursing. It is one thing to explain why partiality in nursing is important, but it is quite another to justify when nurses are permitted to be partial. One possible way of addressing this latter issue evolves from Sarah Stroud's account of permissible partiality.

Stroud's (2010) point is that we are far from impartial in living our daily lives, and this goes for professionals as well. Very often, we advance one person's interests in a way that we do not advance another's (equally important or more important) interests. Stroud's main argument is that some of our choices should be morally protected from what would otherwise be moral demands.

According to Stroud, the reasons for regarding these choices as protected are independent of whatever reasons there may be to demand such behaviour of the agents. Hence, she makes an important distinction between partiality as morally required (e.g. as special partial obligations towards one's child or one's friend) and partiality as morally permitted. Stroud is only interested in the latter, which also has a wider scope than the former. But even though Stroud states that she is interested in an argumentative strategy that does not depend on 'the personal point of view', her position nevertheless falls under this umbrella. I will claim that her arguments might accommodate partiality in nursing, and that this account might be even more reliable than Stroud's original approach.

According to Stroud, our goals, aims, and projects have a special significance to us and thus should be protected from impartial moral demands. They are parts of what Williams called 'an agent's subjective motivational set', your 'S' (Williams, 1981, p. 102). To Williams, one's S is primarily a matter of one's desires (not necessarily egoistic desires). But to Stroud, one's S also includes one's patterns of emotional reactions, personal loyalties, and various projects (Stroud, 2010). There is an important distinction, Stroud says, between a mere preference (i.e. a wish or a want) and a specific goal, aim, or project. A goal is something one *intends to bring about*. It is something towards which one directs agency (i.e. time and energy) (Stroud, 2010). By restricting one's S this way, Stroud wants to avoid the problem of a capacious scope of moral permission.

Stroud's argument for permissible partiality reads as follows:

> Moral demands are, by definition, addressed to *agents*: anything that is subject to a moral demand is, necessarily, an agent. Since morality is necessarily addressed to agents, it seems plausible that it must reflect the *nature* of agents. Here is one pertinent fact about agents: they have projects. (This seems a conceptual, or anyway a necessary, truth about agents.) Furthermore, an agent's projects are necessarily of special significance to him: for me to have something as a project *is* for me to be focusing my energies on it in a way I am not doing for other perhaps equally meritorious pursuits. To ask agents not to do this would be to ask them not to be agents. Morality, then, must not make such a demand; it must, rather, recognize the special significance to agents of their own projects, and permit them to accord those projects special weight. Otherwise it implicitly denies their status as agents.
>
> (Stroud, 2010, pp. 142–143)

This argumentative strategy can also be used with reference to a broader conception of an agent's S. For instance, one might say that (all) agents have things they prefer or care about. They have relationships, preferences for certain hobbies, etc. Stroud's argumentative strategy appears more secure since it allows for a narrower and slimmer definition of the S. One might therefore expect that an *even* slimmer and narrower structure is even more secure. Such a structure arises for instance if the agent's projects are restricted to his projects *as a nurse*. Based on Stroud's structure, we can establish an argument for permissible partiality that corresponds with nurses and nurses' projects: Moral demands of nursing ethics are, by definition, addressed to nurses. Therefore, it seems plausible that such demands must reflect the role of nurses. A pertinent fact about the role of nurses is that they have specific projects. Moreover, a nurse's projects are necessarily of special significance to the nurse *as a nurse*.[3] To ask nurses not to focus their energies on their projects as nurses would be to ask them not to be nurses. Nursing ethics, then, must not make such a demand. It must, rather, recognise the special significance of nurses' projects, and permit them to accord those projects special weight. Otherwise it implicitly denies their status as nurses.

The project in question here should be seen in light of the role-relative obligations nurses are committed to. In Chapter 2 it was argued that members of the nursing profession pursue the collective good represented by their four basic areas of responsibility. These rather generally formulated obligations, which refer to any nursing care activity aimed at meeting a patient's nursing care needs, are discharged in different nursing projects. Any nursing project takes place in relational proximity to the patient, and nurses have a role-relative obligation to accomplish any such project in an adequate and individualised way. Hence, when it is argued that nurses should be allowed to devote time and energy to their project, this is not only aimed at protecting their status as nurses. It is also, and this is perhaps even more important, aimed at protecting the individual patient who is an indispensable part of the project in question.[4] This is why nurses, in some situations, should be permitted to be partial. Otherwise the nurse cannot discharge their professional commitment to patients.

We should note that Stroud's argument only appeals to the agent's own projects, and other people (and their interests and needs) must be a part of the agent's project if it should be protected. The only way, for instance, advancing your welfare should receive some deference from other moral claims on me, Stroud (2010) says, is if it were one of my projects to be doing so. This also means that if advancing your welfare is *not* one of my projects, then my doing so would not receive any protection from otherwise moral concerns. I might of course still advance your welfare, but there is no 'protected zone' for me doing so. Hence, if advancing your welfare is not my project, other moral demands might very well trump my permissibility to do so. And conversely, if providing for a distant patient's nursing care needs (say, for instance, a patient on a waiting list) is not a part of a nurse's project, then morality does not require it. If this is correct, we have the controversial and incredibly problematic conclusion that partiality might surpass the nurse's *permissibility* to provide nursing care to a distant patient. I will not argue for this.

Still, I will argue that relational proximity has some normative significance since it is an essential feature of a nursing project. In Chapter 2 I described partiality in these lines: A patient is given preference over other patient(s) for the reason of relational proximity between the nurse and this patient. I have also argued that partiality in nursing care cannot be based on the non-instrumental value of relationships alone, neither on a premise of a pre-existing partial standing between the nurse and the patient. Instead, it should include a particular understanding of proximity between nurse and patient. The argument for permissible partiality is based on a conception of relational proximity that also incorporates physical and temporal proximity. The nurse,[5] the relevant nursing care, and the patient are all inseparable parts of a particular project. A nursing project, then, can only be carried out when there is a relational proximity between nurse and patient.[6] This is a trivial point, one may say. But relational proximity is what makes the nurse able to sensibly grasp the patient's situation and his or her nursing care needs. This is important, because it requires time and contextual sensitivity, combined with professional knowledge, to perceive the many facets of a patient's nursing care needs. Relational proximity is also an inevitable part of what makes it possible for a nurse to provide adequate nursing care according to perceived needs, thereby discharging the professional responsibility of nursing. But it is important for my discussion at this point to emphasise that relational proximity should not be considered as a physical and quantifiable issue. It should not be conceived of as something that can be measured in minutes or metres. Relational proximity doesn't need to be a face-to-face encounter. As part of a nursing project, it can be, for instance, when a nurse, as part of a rehabilitation programme, phones a patient at home. Relational proximity can also be the face-to-face encounter between the nurse and a patient in an emergency ward. And it can be relational proximity in a more personal sense, as in long-term care:

> In long term caring relationships, personal attachments, and bonds between nurses and their patients may have deep personal significance to the professional carers themselves. The quality and depth of such caring relationships often determine the success of patients' recovery from disease.
>
> (Nortvedt et al., 2011, p. 197)[7,8]

The common feature of relational proximity is that without it, a nursing project cannot be accomplished and the nurse cannot discharge the professional commitment to this particular patient. In other words, relational proximity actualises/symbolises a nurse's commitment to performing the nursing project in an adequate and individualised way.

An important dimension in Stroud's project-based approach to justifying partiality is our relationships (including for instance relationships between spouses, parent and child, friends, and a professor and her students). Stroud's point is that we do not so much put extra weight on these peoples' interests and conferring benefits on them. But we devote our agency to these relationships and to the specific activities they consist of (Stroud, 2010, p. 145). And what is even more important in Stroud's argument is that a fundamental element of these relationships is joint participation. In this sense, it is often a collective or plural activity between agents. Stroud claims that this co-agency has moral significance and may be germane to permissible partiality.

But we do not need a relationship-based premise when the argument is applied to nursing. Stroud's strategy seems to depend on agent-relative reasons explaining the importance of projects to the agent herself. But a nursing project arises from a concern for certain patients (and their interests and needs), and nurses devote their agency to patients as an inevitable part of this project. If they have permission to direct their agency towards their projects, they should also have permission to devote their agency to their patients. The first is not possible without the latter, and vice versa. This notion is of importance both to the nurse (as the agent) and to the patient.

Stroud acknowledges two shortcomings with the project-based account. First, the approach seems only to apply within the contexts of joint agency. In other words, the special moral permissions concern only the project, not any interest of the co-agent outside of this project (Stroud, 2010).

At first glance, this critique is an important one for nursing projects. The moral permission to be partial towards a particular patient is somewhat restricted by his or her need for medical and nursing care. A nurse is not permitted to be partial to the patient's interests outside the context of the particular project. This would mean, for instance, that a district nurse is permitted to favour a patient's need for dressing a wound that is caused by poorly regulated diabetes. But the nurse is not permitted to take into consideration a concern for the patient's financial position which – let us say – may be an underlying source for this patient being unable to regulate his diabetes (with less money, for example, the patient may be limited in his or her ability to buy healthy food). This rationale applies here because finances are not part of the nursing project, whereas dressing a wound is. But to claim this is in some sense to misperceive what nursing care is about. Nursing care must involve some regard for the patient's overall good (but it is not all-encompassing, like parenthood, for example), and a sense of how the good of the caring activity fits into the receiver's overall good, as was one of the arguments in Chapter 2. Hence, Stroud's problem here does not necessarily challenge my account of partiality. This is so because the patient himself, along with the wider scope of the patient's needs, is inevitably a part of a nurse's project. There is then no need for an additional premise of joint agency.

The second problem arising from Stroud's project-based approach is that it might disqualify attachments to persons who cannot participate in joint agency (Stroud, 2010). The quintessential example here is parents' devotion to their newborn child. Since a newborn is not an agent, a relationship like this does not qualify easily for inclusion in the category of shared agency. And the same goes for attachments between two persons who both are agents but where the relationship between them no longer involves shared agency. This might be the case with grown children and parents who live far away from each other, or for old friends living far away from each other (Stroud, 2010). I have already argued that permissible partiality in the context of nursing does not depend on an account of joint agency. The patient is a part of the project because he or she is in need of nursing care. Nursing care is directed to patients, whether or not the patient is an agent (i.e. actively participating in the project). The nursing project has a wide scope. It may be directed at unconscious patients, patients with severe dementia, or any patient who for some reason cannot participate in shared agency.

Here there arises a similarity between Stroud's position and Scheffler's notion of an 'agent-centred prerogative'. In short, Scheffler describes an agent-centred prerogative as follows: 'It would systematically permit people, within certain limits, to devote energy and attention to their projects and commitments even if their doing so would *not* on balance promote the best outcomes overall' (Scheffler, 1982/1994, p. 17). Now, Stroud rejects the agent-centred prerogative as a satisfying way of justifying partiality. Stroud's main critique of agent-centred prerogative is that it protects one's own interests, as a 'partiality to oneself' (Stroud, 2010, p. 137).

But Stroud's objection seems to be premised on a view that does not take professional contexts into consideration. In particular, this regards the premise of joint agency, which, as I argued, does not always apply in nursing care. Basically, this is why I find Stroud's critique of the agent-centred prerogative unsuccessful. To the contrary, her position actually seems to correspond with such a prerogative. Notably, the principal concern in professional care is always for the patient, not for oneself. The upshot of an agent-centred prerogative in nursing is a protection of both the interests of the nurse and the patient.

Scheffler developed his notion of an agent-centred prerogative as a part of his rejection of consequentialism. Although the prerogative aims at protecting the agent's integrity by restricting the requirement of promoting best overall outcomes, such protection is not unlimited. For instance, there cannot be predefined limits to when and how one's interests should be protected:

> That is, it could not reasonably function by requiring each agent to produce the best states of affairs (say) fifty per cent of the time, but releasing him from this requirement for the other fifty per cent of the time and permitting him to do anything whatsoever. This schizophrenic arrangement would, for moral purposes, divide each person into two: a perfect egoist and a perfect consequentialist.
>
> (Scheffler, 1982/1994, p. 17)

Therefore, according to Scheffler, the prerogative is limited to desirable values and activities. It would not be uncontroversial to claim that adequate and individualised nursing care (i.e. any nursing project) is such a desirable value. The aim of a prerogative for partiality in nursing is therefore not to protect the nurse's self-interest (as Scheffler's argument may be taken to imply). It is rather a prerogative to protect values that are desirable for both the nurse and patients.

Importantly then, a prerogative does not permit one to pursue one's projects at all cost. There is a limitation also with regard to the interests of other people. But, Scheffler says,

> a plausible agent-centered prerogative would allow each agent to assign a certain proportionally greater weight to his own interests than to the interests of other people. It would then allow the agent to promote the non-optimal outcome of his choosing, provided only that the degree of its inferiority to each of the superior outcomes he could instead promote in no case exceeded, by more than the specified proportion, the degree of sacrifice necessary for him to promote the superior outcome. If all of the non-optimal outcomes available to the agent were ruled out on these grounds, then and only then would he be required to promote the best overall outcome.
>
> (Scheffler, 1982/1994, p. 20)

This could be taken to imply that a nurse cannot be expected to distribute his or her resources impartially, to the overall good of all patients, if this compromises the desirable value inherent in nursing care (in a nursing project). This is why nurses in some situations should be permitted to be partial to a patient with whom the nurse is relationally close, i.e. with whom she has an ongoing nursing project. If nurses in some situations are not permitted to be partial in this sense, they cannot discharge their professional commitment of providing adequate and individualised nursing care. But as said previously, impartial considerations of distributive justice, etc., could lead to greater professional self-sacrifice when nurses are unable to perform their tasks and discharge the responsibilities to their patients. An important question here concerns the limits or extension of our moral responsibilities with regard to individualised patient care as compared to demands raised by distributive justice, accounting for the needs of non-identified individuals. To include as part of our moral responsibility all moral claims that lie beyond what we directly can control expands moral responsibility to an unlimited extent. For instance, a utilitarian claim that there is no moral difference in your responsibility for an action that you directly caused and an action that you failed to prevent (Scheffler, 2001) has consequences for the way we conceive nurses' professional responsibility.

But before I turn to a discussion of these issues, let me briefly recapitulate that partiality means that in some situations, nurses are permitted to be partial, otherwise he or she cannot discharge the professional commitment. This is a prerogative for permissible partiality. Partiality cannot be a requirement, or a moral duty,[9] since nurses also always have to take impartial considerations into account. For the rest of this chapter, and in Chapter 6, I discuss limits as to when partiality is legitimate and when it is not.

Consequentialism and role-relativity

Scheffler's account of a prerogative bears some resemblance to two out of three types of agent-relative reasons singled out by Nagel. Nagel distinguishes between three reasons that are relative to the moral agent and that in different ways might be protected from impartial moral claims. These are termed by Nagel as 'reasons of autonomy', 'deontological reasons', and 'reasons of obligations' (Nagel, 1986, p. 165). The first category stems from one's desires, projects, commitments, and personal ties to the agent. These reasons serve the agent's own ends; they are optional, and limit what we are obligated to do from an impartial perspective. Since these types of reasons are very much tied to the agent's own personal preferences and desires, this category does not fit well in a professional ethical framework, and I will not discuss it here.

It is the third category identified by Nagel, reasons stemming from one's relationships, which is usually connected with partiality. These 'reasons of obligation' stem from special obligations to closely related persons. The classical examples are relations in families and between friends, but Nagel also includes relations between members of a society or a nation. Such reasons are generated by non-contractual relationships, and resemble Scheffler's 'associative duties' (or special responsibilities). Previously I argued that relationship-based arguments for partiality in nursing care are delicate ones. That is, my claim is that even if some professional relationships can be valued non-instrumentally, this is not the general rule. Additionally, non-instrumental valuing *might* cause arbitrary or biased (illegitimate) partiality if personal or private bonds cause this non-instrumental valuing and, by extension, partiality. And third, it is unreasonable to expect any nurse (or patient) to value any professional relationship non-instrumentally. I do not deny that in some cases partiality in nursing care might be justified on relationship-based reasons, but it seems implausible to base an argument for the normative significance of partiality on such a requirement alone.

It should be clear by now that reasons for partiality in nursing care should not be based on any personal or private bonds or relations between the nurse and the patient (or his/her relatives). I have also argued that to the extent that agent-relativity matters normatively in nursing, we are dealing with *role*-relativity and not agent-relativity in a personal sense. Other-directedness, as concern for the patient's subjective and objective needs, is an indispensable part of a nursing project. To be normatively significant in nursing care, agent-centredness must incorporate other-direction.

Based on this background, and for the purpose of justifying partiality in nursing care, my interest in Nagel's second category of agent-relative restrictions arose. These are the deontological agent-relative constraints. In short, these are constraints on an agent's action that arise from the right of others not to be harmed. In the next chapter I want to explore such arguments, especially with regard to the questions of partiality and justice in nursing care. In order to refer these arguments to their contexts, I will start out with a brief presentation of consequentialism. Needless to say, I cannot capture the innumerable amount of literature on consequentialism. My ambition is to present the main features of consequentialism and the most widespread objections to it.

Partiality, consequentialism, and role-relativity

Until now I have only briefly touched upon consequentialism. As maximising health-related benefit is a central macro-level value in health care, utilitarianism/consequentialism proves to be a central approach to distributing health care resources. Interestingly, an influential critique of utilitarianism focuses on its lack of concern for fairness in distributive justice (Scheffler, 1988; Rawls, 1971). On the other hand, there are also considerable discussions in moral philosophy on the relation between consequentialism and agent-relativity.[10]

The term 'consequentialism' is sometimes used interchangeably with the term 'utilitarianism'. A more common view is to consider utilitarianism as *a version of* consequentialism. Others, such as Timothy Chappell, use the term 'consequentialism' in a more narrow sense as being *a part of* utilitarianism. Chappell defines utilitarianism as consistent with the four components maximalism, welfarism, aggregationism, and consequentialism, where the latter tells us that the best is 'a state of affairs, a set of consequences, that is achievable by action' (Chappell, 2009, p. 127).

The most significant message from consequentialism is that the consequences of any relevant alternative should be ranked from best to worst from an impersonal and impartial point of view. And then the agent should choose the act that has the best consequences. In utilitarian terms this means to increase happiness or pleasure or welfare for the greatest number, and/or to minimise negative consequences for the greatest number. Consequentialism in general is only concerned with consequences and the maximisation of utility. Hence, there is an important sense in which impartiality in consequentialism is concerned neither about equality[11] nor the individuality of persons.

A point of departure for my discussion here is Scheffler's remark that consequentialism comes in two parts. First, 'it gives some principle for ranking overall states of affairs from best to worst from an impersonal standpoint' (Scheffler, 1988, p. 1), and second, 'it says that the right act in any given situation is the one that will produce the highest-ranked state of affairs that the agent is in a position to produce' (Scheffler, 1988, p. 1). Whereas objections to consequentialism are seldom directed at the first part of Scheffler's definition, the target of most critics is the second part. According to Scheffler, non-consequentialists typically object in two ways to this part. First, one may be forbidden to do a certain thing that may result in the best overall outcome (Scheffler, 1988), because one is under obligation to perform another act. This objection refers to agent-relative *restrictions*. Later in this chapter I discuss one such restriction, i.e. deontological restrictions. Agent-relative *deontological* restrictions are essentially a constraint on what an agent is *permitted* to do. But I will also argue that an agent-relative restriction may work as a restriction on what an agent should be required to do. A second objection argues that one is not required to do the thing that produces the best overall outcome (Scheffler, 1988) Often it is up to the individual agent to decide whether one is so required. Besides, since, as Scheffler argues, that morality leaves people some freedom of choice, sometimes one may want to do the thing that produces the best overall outcome, and sometimes not (Scheffler, 1988). This objection refers to agent-relative *permissions*, or what Scheffler calls an agent-relative *prerogative.*

There are in particular two challenging claims of consequentialism that have provoked criticism. One is that it requires people to do any act that will produce the best overall outcome (Scheffler, 1988), and further that it is an extremely demanding moral theory since it requires a neglect of one's pursuit whenever one instead could do something that could produce slightly more good (Scheffler, 1988) Another influential and well-known critic of consequentialism, Bernard Williams (1973), argues that the demands of consequentialism undermine the integrity of the individual. His critique mainly applies to this second challenging claim of consequentialism. Williams's argument in this context is that to always think impartially about one's attachments, personal projects, and relationships, tends to undermine a person's integrity, his or her sense of self, and even his or her humanity. Unfortunately, then, the individual care worker seems to be obligated to have 'one thought too many' (Williams, 1981, p. 18). That is, even though it can be argued – as I did in the previous section – that nurses might have a prerogative for partiality, impartial concern for the good of each patient must always be a part of the judgment. In an article from 2008 on the normative significance of proximity in ethics, Nortvedt and myself argued that from the perspective of Williams, jeopardising professional ethics and values intrinsic to nursing will undermine the care worker's integrity (Nortvedt and Nordhaug, 2008). But as should be clear by now, arguments for partiality in nursing care should incorporate the perspective of the patients. In the next section I discuss how the rights of other persons are an indispensible part of role-relative constraints. For instance, the right not to be maltreated or harmed might correspond with an agent's obligation not to maltreat or harm anyone.

Partiality and deontological role-relative constraints

Earlier in this chapter I discussed the agent-centred prerogative for partiality in nursing care. This is a restriction regarding the permissibility of actions. But the discussions above also brought in another type of agent-relative restriction, namely, that of deontological restrictions. One way of understanding a deontological restriction in nursing care is as a principle of not harming. As demonstrated earlier, principle is also emphasised in care ethics. That is, at least the principle is not incompatible with care ethics. The principle appears, however, to be incompatible with consequentialism. Anyway, agent-centred deontological restrictions are initially constraints on what an agent is permitted to do. And these restrictions most often affect the consequentialistic principle of utility maximisation where the end justifies the means. A more moderate restriction is found in Scheffler's hybrid model of an agent-centred prerogative (see the section 'A prerogative of partiality in nursing', above). Here, the agent is permitted to act out of consequentialistic concerns, but should also be permitted a so-called 'protected zone' for his or her valuable projects (or relationships).

Deontological constraints, Thomas Nagel says, do not depend on the agent's projects and aims, but on the claims of others (Nagel, 1986). Agent-relative reasons of deontology stem from the claim of others not to be maltreated. Let us take a look at a passage where Nagel exemplifies a deontological agent-centred restriction:

> You have an auto accident one winter night on a lonely road. The other passengers are badly injured, the car is out of commission, and the road is deserted, so you run along it till you find an isolated house. The house turns out to be occupied by an old woman who is looking after her small grandchild. There is no phone, but there is a car in the garage, and you ask desperately to borrow it, and explain the situation. She doesn't believe you. Terrified by your desperation she runs upstairs and locks herself in the bathroom, leaving you alone with the child. You pound ineffectively on the door and search without success for the car keys. Then it occurs to you that she might be persuaded to tell you where they are if you were to twist the child's arm outside the bathroom door. Should you do it? It is difficult not to see this as a dilemma, even though the child's getting its arm twisted is a minor evil compared with your friends' not getting to the hospital. The dilemma must be due to a special reason against *doing* such a thing. Otherwise it would be obvious that you should choose the lesser evil and twist the child's arm.
>
> (Nagel, 1986, p. 176)

Reasons of deontology limit what we are permitted to do and are therefore also termed agent-centred restrictions. According to Scheffler (1982/1994) a deontological restriction would typically be directed to the agent's obligation to act out of impartial consequentialistic concerns. Scheffler describes these restrictions as

> restrictions on action which have the effect of denying that there is any non-agent-relative principle for ranking overall states of affairs from best to worst such that it is always permissible to produce the best available state of affairs so characterized.
>
> (Scheffler, 1982/1994, pp. 2–3)

The classic target then for this kind of restriction is the consequentialist claim that killing one innocent person is permissible (even required) if (and only if) this is the only way to prevent the death of two (or more) other innocent people. The reason for why this is wrong, according to deontology, refers back to other people's right not to be maltreated (for instance, not being killed when you are innocent). Conversely, an agent cannot be required to maltreat other people (for instance to kill an innocent person), and from such reasoning arises a deontological agent-relative restriction. This is an interesting restriction for the partialist–impartialist debate in nursing. Consider a consequentialist claim that the right thing to do is to neglect or compromise one patient's need for nursing care since such neglect would make it possible to provide nursing care to two (or more) other patients. It seems absurd to act upon such a line of reasoning. And it also seems absurd to *require* nurses to compromise a patient's need on such reasoning.[12] Nagel finds such deontological agent-centred constraints very puzzling because of the essentiality of the particular relation of the agent to the outcome (1986). And while Nagel doubts that any of the three types of agent-relative reasons really exist, he places more weight on the two former categories than on the third.

For the purpose of justifying partiality in nursing care, however, the focus on other-centredness convinced me that the third category (i.e. reasons of obligation) could prove to be constructive. And perhaps, in some sense, deontological agent-centred restrictions are less difficult to explain in relation to professionals simply because professionals are (by definition) subordinated to duties that are also action-guiding. This is not so in our ordinary, private lives. But even now, the tricky question is how deontological reasons in fact motivate. And it definitively does not explain why the reason is agent-relative and not agent-neutral. The reason for not neglecting a patient's need for nursing care applies to any nurse, not just to a particular nurse. However, this general constraint does not apply to just anyone. If you are not a nurse, then you cannot appeal to this particular deontological restriction.

The reason for not neglecting a patient's need for nursing care is not an agent-neutral reason that pertains to anyone; one must be a nurse to have such a reason. And one must be a patient with a (legitimate) need for nursing care to have the corresponding right of not having these needs neglected.[13] Deontological reasons in nursing care are not agent-neutral in a universal sense, and neither are the values behind them. They are rather role-relative. But this does not explain Nagel's worry. I have simply said that in nursing, there may be deontological restrictions that only apply to nurses. No nurse is permitted to neglect a patient's need for nursing care (as no person is permitted to twist a child's arm). The question of interest is whether they are reasons or restrictions that apply to particular nurses (in particular situations) or to any nurse (as role-relativity formulated in general terms). The normative potential of deontological restrictions or reasons has difficulty explaining whether these are agent-neutral or agent-relative. Agent-neutral deontological reasons apply to me with the same force as if they were agent-relative. Wouldn't the constraint against twisting the child's arm be equally strong independent of it being agent-neutral or agent-relative? Agent-relative reasons apply especially to the agent, but not necessarily with greater normative force than if they are agent-neutral. The reason is the same and the normative significance is independent of them being neutral or relative to the agent to whom they apply. If this is so, the question is how such a deontological constraint can be explained in itself. Or is it? Nagel's query evokes questions of moral realism as well as moral internalism:

> The phenomenological fact to be accounted for is that we seem to apprehend in each individual case an extremely powerful agent-relative *reason* not to harm an innocent person. This presents itself as the apprehension of a normative truth, not just as a psychological inhibition.
>
> (Nagel, 1986, p. 179)

Without going into discussions of the meta-ethical issues of moral realism, subjectivism, or the relation between internalism and externalism in ethics,[14] I suggest that the phenomenological fact Nagel perhaps stresses best can be comprehended within the frame of moral realism.[15]

A possible explanation from the moral realism of agent-relativity would be to take as a departure that pain exists as a normative fact, and as something to be relieved and avoided. According to Nortvedt these are 'moral properties that exist independent of subjective perception and evaluation' (Nortvedt, 2012, p. 2). How this can be so, and how the perception of a moral reality motivates action, are questions I leave open. The point here is that if moral realism is correct, it has the potential to explain (and perhaps also justify) how the perception of the person(s) injured in the car accident in Nagel's example gave you a reason for saving them.[16] The point here is that an agent-relative reason exists here and now, because it is you – and no one else – who is there and able to perceive the injured persons.[17] Nagel uses the words 'saving your friends', but the fact that the injured persons are your friends is irrelevant for the reason's creation. Anyone in the same situation would have the same reason, but it is the person confronted with the need who is able to do something about it. Furthermore, if moral realism is correct, our 'intuition' that preventing pain is the right thing to do must be explained. Twisting the child's arm is to inflict pain on someone, and it is counterintuitive to do so – not because of some calculation of consequences (getting the car keys and saving the injured persons), but because you put yourself in a situation where more pain will arise. There is a constraint on the agent who is confronted with the possibility of inflicting pain that could and should be avoided. Perhaps a deontological restriction arises from someone's claim not to be maltreated, and from the agent's own resistance against being confronted with even more pain. One question regarding agent-neutrality and agent-relativity is how and why someone perceives pain (and other moral realties if they exist) as a reason for action, and others not. Maybe this is also what makes the distinction regarding deontological constraints puzzling.

Now, recall Nagel's example of one's resistance to twisting a child's arm even if it could prevent some greater harm. There is an agent-neutral value behind the intuition of not wanting to twist a child's arm. But there is an agent-relative reason behind the resistance, Nagel says, 'because the particular relation of the agent to the outcome is essential' (Nagel, 1986, p. 176). Deontological restrictions do not rely on some personal connection between the nurse and the patient. That is, such restrictions do not presuppose a non-instrumental valuing of the relationship or a non-instrumental valuing of the 'nursing project'. Rather, it is a restriction that applies to any nurse confronted with (for instance) the maximising claims of consequentialism. In the context of nursing care, then, the restriction implies that no nurse should be required to act out of such consequentialist concerns because all patients have a right to not be neglected. Even more to the point, a deontological restriction implies that no nurse is *permitted* to neglect or compromise a patient's need for nursing care for the sake of providing nursing care to other patients. This must be seen in relation to the impartial duties and principles that inform deontological restrictions. For instance, a principle of beneficence and a principle of not harming represent professional duties relevant for nursing care. These duties are general in that they apply to any nurse, regardless of who the patient is. Hence, a nurse cannot appeal to a principle of not harming as a deontological restriction based on the reason that 'it is my patient'. In this particular sense, a deontological agent-centred restriction does not qualify as a reason for partiality. But in particular cases, a nurse's concern for a particular patient might trump her concern for other patients on certain conditions. Such conditions are found in Scheffler's description of an agent-centred restriction:

> An agent-centered restriction is, roughly, a restriction which it is at least sometimes impermissible to violate in circumstances where a violation would serve to minimize total overall violations of the very same restriction, and would have no other morally relevant consequences.
> (Scheffler, 1988, p. 243)

Consider the restriction of neglecting a patient's need. Two conditions must, then, according to Scheffler, be satisfied. First, (at least sometimes) it is impermissible to neglect a patient's need in circumstances where neglecting this patient's need would serve to minimise the neglect of other patients' needs. The premise here seems to be that the principle (or rule or some other general or universal deontological concern) that the agent should act from is the same principle that might be violated if she or he does not act from this principle. Hence, the first condition could also be expressed as such: (at least sometimes) it is not permissible to violate the principle of x if (or even if) the violation of x would serve to minimise the total overall violation of x. Compromising a patient's need is an act of harm. And *principally* the nurse has a duty not to harm a patient, and therefore not neglect a patient's need. The question of interest here is how this relates to partiality. It follows from this first condition that a nurse cannot apply to the principle of beneficence as a reason for partiality if this breaks a different principle, say the principle of not harming (causes harm to other patients). But it also follows that (at least sometimes) the nurse is permitted to apply to the principle of beneficence as a reason for partiality even if it breaks the principle of beneficence towards other patients. As regards partiality there might be a deontological restriction for a nurse to compromise one patient's need to the benefit of other patients. But this is of course a delicate argument, since the duty not to harm relates to all patients. Needs assessments are therefore necessary to avoid arbitrary or biased partiality.

The second condition in Scheffler's definition is that the restriction would have no other morally relevant consequences. It should go without saying that what counts as morally relevant consequences will vary from case to case. But it is nevertheless important that patients' medical needs and needs for nursing care are part of this judgment. In Chapter 6 I explore and discuss how needs assessments could play a part in the partiality–justice debate.

Concluding remarks

Once the challenges of care ethics were discussed in the previous chapter, I turned to the other position that underscores the moral value of relational concerns. I began exploring Scheffler's arguments for the normative significance of interpersonal relationships. Scheffler's main argument is – in short – that as long as interpersonal relationships are valued non-instrumentally, they generate reasons for partiality between the parties in the valued relationship. Moreover, such a reason for partiality cannot (always) be ruled out by reasons for impartiality. It turned out, however, that the key problem when applying Scheffler's normative argument for partiality to nursing care relates to its main premise. That is, Scheffler argues that it is the non-instrumental valuing of a relationship that generates reasons for partiality. But in nursing care, one cannot and should not expect a non-instrumental valuing of the relation between a nurse and a patient. This is so because the existence of a professional caring relationship is based on objective and/or subjective *needs* of nursing care. Therefore, the professional relationship is mainly of an instrumental character. I do not dismiss the idea that sometimes a nurse and a patient actually value the relationship non-instrumentally. And I am also sympathetic to the idea that they sometimes *should* value it non-instrumentally. Indeed, a non-instrumental valuing of a professional relationship might even have a therapeutic effect (which, of course, is to say that a non-instrumental valuing might be a means for an instrumental purpose). Nevertheless, in general, the *premise* of non-instrumental valuing makes Scheffler's partial position difficult to apply to a professional context. Then I turned from relationship-based approaches to a more project-based approach to partiality. Inspired by Stroud's account of permissible partiality and Scheffler's prerogative for partiality, I aimed to establish an argument for a prerogative of partiality within the nursing project. This prerogative should be seen as a means to protect both the interests of the nurse (and the nursing profession that possesses the mandate of providing nursing care) and the interest of the patient(s). The prerogative can also be seen in light of Nagel's account of deontological restrictions. Such a restriction can be taken to protect individuals both from being maltreated or harmed and from being required to maltreat or harm – even if maltreating and harming could prevent even greater maltreatment and harming of others. As for the question of partiality, we could say that there might be a restriction on compromising a patient's needs for nursing care, even if this could benefit others. But since the restriction on compromising needs relates to any patient, any decision concerning partiality and impartiality must take needs assessments into account.

So far, my argument for partiality can briefly be summarised as follows: Nursing care is the desirable collective good pursued by the nursing profession. This collective good is represented by the four general patient-centred areas of responsibility, i.e. promoting health, preventing illness, restoring health, and alleviating suffering. Any patient-centred caring activity in nursing can be conceptualised within the umbrella term of the 'nursing project'. All projects of nursing take place in some form of relational proximity between a nurse and a patient.[18] Then, situational circumstances, such as resource constraints, along with claims of impartiality, sometimes limit nurses' ability to discharge or fulfil a nursing project. This may prevent nurses from pursuing the collective good to which they are obligated. This is why we need a normative argument for partiality in nursing care. I have based my discussion and argument on the following account of partiality: Partiality means that one patient is given precedence over another based on relational proximity. My justification of partiality takes as its departure role-relative reasons, along with reasons from the care receiver's perspective (such as the right not to be harmed or maltreated). The nursing project then is a relational project, where both the nurse and the patient are indispensable parts. To compromise this project is to compromise both nurses and patients. Therefore, I aimed to develop a prerogative for protecting a nursing project. Or to put it more to the point, a prerogative aimed at protecting nursing care that takes place in relational proximity between nurse and patient. This prerogative states that nurses who are committed to a nursing project sometimes are permitted to be partial. Relational proximity to a patient is an indispensable part of this project, and embodies the ongoing project. So far, two deontological restrictions on the prerogative for partiality have been established: (1) a nurse might not be permitted to neglect a patient's needs even if doing so would minimise harm to other patients, and (2) a nurse might have a restriction against breaking a principle of beneficence to a patient even if doing so could serve to maximise beneficence to other patients. In the next chapter I discuss another important and interrelated restriction on permissible partiality, namely that of needs assessments.

Notes

1 Scheffler also labels these responsibilities 'associative duties'. In this way, Scheffler can be taken to signify that we are not only permitted to act from our special responsibilities, but sometimes we are obligated to do so.

2 Of course, Mary might value the relationship with Tom non-instrumentally independently of this – because, say, she happens to like Tom personally, and therefore also feels comfortable and safe in his company. If so, this emotional attachment should be seen as one of Mary's subjective needs and therefore also an important part of Tom's nursing project responsibilities to Mary. This non-instrumental valuing may even have a therapeutic effect. But Mary (as a patient) cannot and should not be expected to have any special responsibility to Tom (as a nurse). Although Scheffler does not explicitly address the issues of reciprocity and special obligations in asymmetrical caring relationships, it seems reasonable to assume from his position that special responsibility only arises when the *caregiver* values the relationship non-instrumentally.

3 Note that this does not presuppose that a nurse values the project non-instrumentally.

4 If we recall the distinctions made in Chapter 2 between subject-giving reasons and object-giving reasons for partiality, the argument above resembles a subject-giving (general), role-relative reason for partiality. That is, it is an argument premised on the perspective of the agent, not the care receiver (or 'object'). Although I maintain that partiality might be of importance for nurses, and even for the nursing profession, an argument for partiality in nursing care should primarily be established on behalf of – and for the sake of – the patients. This is what in Chapter 2 I called object-giving reasons. Since, however, nursing care is and must be relational, subject-giving and object-giving reasons for partiality overlap.

5 Previously I have discussed whether a nurse is replaceable with another nurse. He or she might be, but that shouldn't alter the idea of a nursing project. What I am arguing for is a protection of a nursing project, not a particular nurse's project. So when I also argue for the protection of the nurse's integrity, this is an argument on behalf of any nurse.

6 Let me remind the reader that here I am only concerned about nursing care at clinical levels, where concrete caring activities take place.

7 See also Nortvedt (1996).

8 This resembles the way Scheffler argues for special obligation for the reason of non-instrumental valuing of a relationship. As I said in the discussion of Scheffler's position above, I do not object that such valuing exists in professional relationships. But my point was that this cannot be the main reason for professional partiality.

9 Of course, from this a delicate problem arises since adequate and individualised nursing care can be considered as a patient's right.

10 See for instance Parfit (1984); Dancy (1993); Tännsjö (1995); Scheffler (1982/1994); (1988).

11 The most well-known critique of utilitarianism's ignorance of equality and fairness in the distribution of goods stems from John Rawls (1971).

12 It is dubious whether there is any normative reason for compromising or neglecting a patient's need for nursing care. In cases of priority, attention to severe medical conditions should certainly take precedence over basic nursing care needs, and there should always be a professional assessment of severity of needs of nursing care. But this does not pertain to the total neglect of some needs.

13 Of course, common-sense morality tells us that anyone (either in an agent-neutral or agent-relative way) has reason not to neglect someone in need, and that anyone in need has a right not to be neglected. But it is the regulated particular duty of professionals and the regulated rights of patients I am concerned about here.

14 See for instance Dancy (1993).

15 See for instance Nortvedt (2012) and Tännsjö (2010).
16 We would of course also have a *legal* obligation to save injured persons (and non-human animals) we come across.
17 See Raustøl (2010) for a discussion of acuteness as a reason for partiality.
18 Technological care is an advancing part of present and future health care. Technology that is controlled by someone other than the client, such as GPS tracking of demented patients, as well as client-controlled technological tools, such as security alarms for the elderly, provoke several ethical questions. One such question concerns technology superseding human face-to-face care.

References

Blum, L., 1994. *Moral perception and particularity*. Cambridge: Cambridge University Press.
Chappell, T., 2009. *Ethics and experience: Life beyond moral theory*. Durham, NC: Acumen.
Dancy, J., 1993. *Moral reasons*. Oxford: Blackwell.
Miller, S., 2010. *The moral foundations of social institutions: A philosophical study*. Cambridge: Cambridge University Press.
Nagel, T., 1986. *The view from nowhere*. New York: New York University Press.
Nordhaug, M. and Nortvedt, P., 2011. Justice and proximity: Problems for an ethics of care. *Health Care Analysis*, 19, pp. 3–14.
Nortvedt, P., 1996. *Sensitive judgment: Nursing, moral philosophy and an ethics of care*. Oslo: Tano Aschehoug.
Nortvedt, P., 2012. The normativity of clinical health care: Perspectives on moral realism. *Journal of Medicine and Philosophy*, 37(3), pp. 295–309.
Nortvedt, P., Hem, M. and Skirbekk, H., 2011. The ethics of care: Role obligations and moderate partiality in health care. *Nursing Ethics*, 18(2), pp. 192–200.
Nortvedt, P. and Nordhaug, M., 2008. The principle and problem of proximity in ethics. *Journal of Medical Ethics*, 34(3), pp. 156–161.
Oakley, J. and Cocking, D., 2001. *Virtue ethics and professional roles*. Cambridge: Cambridge University Press.
Parfit, D., 1984. *Reasons and persons*. Oxford: Clarendon Press.
Raustøl, A., 2010. Impartiality and partiality in nursing ethics. s. l. Dissertation, University of Reading.
Rawls, J., 1971. *A theory of justice*. s. l. Cambridge, MA: Harvard University Press.
Scheffler, S., 1982/1994. *The rejection of consequentialism: A philosophical investigation of the considerations underlying rival moral conceptions*. Oxford: Clarendon Press.
Scheffler, S., 1988. Agent-centered restrictions, rationality, and the virtues. In: Scheffler, S., ed., *Consequentialism and its critics*. Oxford: Oxford University Press, pp. 243–260.
Scheffler, S., 2001. *Boundaries and allegiances*. Oxford: Oxford University Press.
Scheffler, S., 2010. *Equality and tradition*. New York: Oxford University Press.
Stroud, S., 2010. Permissible partiality, projects, and plural agency. In: Feltham, B. and Cottingham, J., eds, *Partiality and impartiality: Morality, special relationships, and the wider world*. Oxford: Oxford University Press, pp. 131–150.
Tännsjö, T., 1995. Blameless wrongdoing. *Ethics*, 106(1), pp. 120–127.
Tännsjö, T., 2010. *From reasons to norms*. Dordrecht: Springer.
Williams, B., 1981. *Moral luck*. Cambridge: Cambridge University Press.
Williams, B., 1973. *Problems of the self*. Cambridge: Cambridge University Press.

6 Partiality, justice, and moral dilemmas

In the previous chapter, I described a prerogative for permissible partiality in nursing care. Except for a role-relative restriction against harming patients, the question of which situations should allow partiality remains unanswered. This will be the main topic of this chapter. I will approach these questions by first discussing partiality and impartiality in clinical priority decisions by using the formal principle of justice. In the article 'Justice and Proximity: Problems for an Ethics of Care' (Nordhaug and Nortvedt, 2011) Nortvedt and I discuss partiality and impartiality in light of the formal principle of justice. The first part of this chapter is a further discussion of main points of this article, where relational proximity is applied as a material principle of distributive justice. The principle of formal justice is designed to secure impartiality and consistency in moral deliberations. Subsequently, if a priority decision based on relational proximity is morally legitimate, it cannot be inconsistent with this principle.

An issue that complicates the discussion is the importance of the assessments of patients' medical needs and nursing care needs[1] in priority decisions. As I said in Chapter 3, a nurse ought to give priority to the most severe and urgent needs, but is still committed to respond to other less severe or less urgent needs. Assessments of objective needs are always the initial, fundamental focus of priority decisions, and severity of needs most often takes precedence over other concerns in priority decisions. In Chapter 3 it was argued that as long as the need in question is *occurrent or about to become occurrent*, needs should be prioritised according to a hierarchy where vital needs are the most pressing, followed by needs related to harm and needs related to well-being. Additionally, dispositional needs for nursing care should be prevented from becoming occurrent.

At the same time, I have argued that partiality based on relational proximity might be permissible, and even desirable. But relational proximity to patients and severity of needs do not always coincide. Moreover, in some situations patients have needs that are either of equal severity or are equal in some other morally relevant sense. In the section on 'Partiality and the formal principle of justice', I will argue that partiality is permissible in such situations. As will be shown, this discussion explores some limitations to partiality. But we also are faced with cases that cannot be solved in any principled way; these moral dilemmas will be discussed in the section on 'Partiality, tragic choices, and moral blamelessness'.

I do not intend to find an unambiguous way out of the tensions between partiality and impartiality. In fact, I do not think any simple solution can be found. The best we can hope for is to establish some kind of balance between modest partiality and a modest impartiality,[2] and that balance is what this chapter intends to find. I will bring the chapter to a close by arguing that as long as the partial acts in question are morally permissible, the nurse is morally blameless for the unavoidable consequences for other patients of such partial acts.

Partiality and the formal principle of justice

Relational proximity and the formal principle of justice

The formal principle of justice states that it is unjust to give different treatment to individuals who are alike in every relevant respect, and to give equal treatment to individuals who are different in some relevant respect (Feinberg, 1973). Three clarifications should then be made. First, what counts as a relevant difference? Second, what are the contexts of application? And third, what is the 'treatment' in question? As regards the first clarification, I have already said that needs assessments play a significant role in clinical priority decisions. Hence, 'to each according to need' is an important material principle for distributive justice in nursing care. But for the purpose of legitimating partiality, which is, according to my definition, based on relational proximity rather than particular needs, this is not the material principle we are looking for. Instead, I take needs assessments as considerably important for a discussion of restrictions to permissible partiality. In the previous chapter, I argued that in some situations, a nurse who is committed to a nursing project should be permitted to act partially in this project. Otherwise, the nurse cannot discharge her professional commitment. This argument was based on the presumption that relational proximity is an essential property of a nursing project and plays a fundamental role for nursing care to be exercised adequately and in an individualised way. This is why I suggest 'relational proximity' to function as a material principle for the discussion that follows. Therefore, I take relational proximity to imply that a relevant difference between patients justifies differential treatment. But notably, relational proximity cannot be decisive independently of needs assessments in concrete caring situations. This implies, as we shall see, that no clear-cut guidelines for permissible partiality can be established.

The second clarification regards the context for applying the material principles. The context of interest here is clinical health care prioritisations. Note that this does not amount to questions of rationalising health care services on an institutional or political level. I am not interested here in superior priority decisions regarding, for instance, hip replacement surgery or heart surgery. Of interest are the daily decisions that nurses at a clinical level have to make, mostly due to scarcity of resources, concerning which patient's needs should be prioritised for care.

As for the third clarification, the 'treatment' in question does not refer to particular, concrete medical treatment or nursing procedures. Hence, the term 'treatment' is somewhat misleading. What it signifies here is partiality based on relational proximity. In other words, the *differential treatment in question concerns adequate time and attention for the patient to whom the nurse is relationally close because of a nursing project.*

There are two main scenarios that result from applying 'relational proximity' as a material criterion. On the one hand, all things considered, if two (or more) patients have equal needs for nursing care and are equally close to the nurse, these patients should be treated equally by the nurse. On the other hand, if two (or more) patients have unequal needs for nursing care and there is inequality regarding relational closeness to the nurse, these patients should be treated unequally (Nordhaug and Nortvedt, 2011). Since the intention is to discuss limits to *permissible* partiality, the use of the verb 'should' here seems mistaken, or (at best) confusing. 'Could' would perhaps be a better word, since I do not think partiality can be morally mandatory. It is indeed challenging to adequately capture the complexities of clinical nursing practice in a theoretical and moral philosophical language. But as the discussion will show, priority decisions must take relevant contextual considerations into account, which means that whether or not one *should* be partial in 'real life' nursing practice will vary from situation to situation.

This raises an important question as to how equality and inequality of relational proximity should be interpreted. Let me remind the reader that, as said in the previous chapter, I do not take relational proximity to be a quantifiable entity. The basic point for my discussion here is that there is a real connection between nurse and patient, and that this connection is what makes the relevant nursing project 'real' and actualises the nurse's commitment to providing adequate and individualised nursing care to this particular patient. Hence, when I go on to discuss equality and inequality in relational proximity, I am not referring to absolute and accurately comparable dimensions. Sometimes there are obvious differences in relational proximity, for instance, as in the example with Mary and the unknown distant patient on the waiting list. There is no (existing) relational proximity between the nurse Tom and the patient on the waiting list, i.e. there is no nursing project established. But there is one between Tom and Mary. In other cases, as when a nurse has several ongoing nursing projects, it becomes difficult or even impossible to discern inequality in relational proximity. This could occur, for instance, when a nurse is responsible for five patients in the same ward.

In what follows I discuss the implications of taking needs assessments into account when 'relational proximity' is the applied material principle of distributive justice. First, I discuss situations where there is equality in needs, and unequal relational proximity. Then I turn to situations where there are unequal needs and unequal relational proximity. And then, finally, I discuss situations where there is equality in relational proximity, combined with equality in needs or inequality in needs, respectively.

Unequal cases should be treated unequally: cases of inequality in relational proximity

The formal principle of justice states that equal cases should be treated equally, and unequal cases should be treated unequally. When applying proximity as a material principle, and there is unequal relational proximity, cases should be treated unequally (with regard to the degree of relational proximity). When accounting for a needs assessment, we obtain two prospects: (1) Equality in need implies no differences between patients. This means that proximity might in some situations be decisive for prioritising.[3] (2) Inequality in need implies a difference between patients. This means that relational proximity cannot work as the single determining factor. I will discuss these two possibilities in turn.

Equality in needs

When there is equality in needs but unequal relational proximity, patients should be treated unequally. This would imply that when there is relational proximity between a nurse and a patient, but not so between the nurse and another patient, and the needs of these two patients are equal, the nurse is permitted to be partial to the former patient.[4] In other words, the nurse is permitted to be partial to the current nursing project. For example, an inpatient in a hospital ward is closer to a nurse working in this ward than a patient waiting for admission to the same ward, and the nurse is therefore permitted to be partial to the needs of the inpatient.

But such a conclusion is valid if, and only if, there is equality in need. It is, however, extremely uncertain whether such cases exist. As Chappell says, there are no qualitatively indiscernible cases, not even in everyday life; there are only cases that are roughly similar (2009).

When needs are comprehended solely as objective needs, it may be easier to compare them. For instance, in general, any patients experiencing cardiac arrest are in (objective) need of life-saving treatment. Hence, in general, they have equal medical needs. And, in general, any patients with bacterial pneumonia are in need of antibiotics. Therefore, in general, any patients with bacterial pneumonia have equal medical needs. But even then it is doubtful whether such equality really exists. This is so because medical decision-making is also fuelled by information that takes into account, for example, the particular patient's co-morbidity and health status, as well as a concern for the patient's subjective analysis of his or her needs and condition. Medical decisions are primarily, but not solely, based on medical criteria. For instance, acute renal failure is a very severe condition and should be prioritised for treatment.

Hence, if two patients are hospitalised for acute renal failure and are offered the same medical treatment, their similarities in needs may very well stop there. It may be that these two patients need *unequal* nursing care even though they are considered equal according to their relevant medical needs. It might very well be the case that, for instance, one of these patients is otherwise healthy and does not need any additional nursing care, whereas the other patient is very anxious about the situation and about leaving the hospital, in need of assistance with his morning toileting and with regard to nutrition, and should not be discharged from the hospital before the community care is ready to take care of him at home. Hence, it is doubtful, but not unthinkable, that cases of *inequality in relational proximity* combined with *equality in needs* exist.

So far I have argued that inequality in relational proximity combined with equality in needs, justifies partiality in a way that is consistent with the formal principle of justice. I also questioned whether equality in needs really exists. But the question of whether or not needs are equal relates, I will argue, to the relative level of need severity or whether the needs are comparable at all. Some needs are more acute and critical than others, or they are simply too different to be compared, but of equal moral relevance. An example of the severity of need situation is the inequality between cardiac arrest and bacterial pneumonia. Cardiac arrest is an acute life-threatening situation where immediate intervention is necessary. Bacterial pneumonia might also be a severe medical condition, but is less acute than cardiac arrest, and the need for immediate intervention is most often not that urgent. An example of situations that are too different to be compared is the inequality between caring for a patient on his deathbed and arranging for a patient's self-care in a rehabilitation unit. These patients' needs are too different to be compared in absolute terms. But they may be of approximately equal moral worth and relevance.

Besides, in clinical health care, situations change during a shift, sometimes quickly, as when a patient's medical condition suddenly goes from bad to worse. Sometimes these changes are less acute, as when new patients arrive at the nursing home or the community nurse has to visit one more patient. In such cases, the nurse is confronted with situations where there is *inequality in need*. I will first consider such situations combined with inequality in relational proximity. Later in this chapter, I turn to cases where inequality in need is combined with *equality in relational proximity*. And then, finally, I discuss cases where there is equality in both relational proximity and need (to the extent that these cases exist).

Inequality in needs

Consider situations where there are severe conditions present, such as cardiac arrest or even bacterial pneumonia. It should go without saying that severe conditions like these should be prioritised for medical intervention and nursing care. It should also go without saying that partiality based on relational proximity to a patient with less severe needs should not trump concern for a more distant patient with more severe needs. For instance, a community nurse performing a morning toileting on a patient should not appeal to the principle of relational proximity if a patient (who, say, lives next door) falls down the stairs and cries out for help. In such a situation, the nurse should of course attend to the crying patient next door. Here we have a situation where the patient with the less severe need is relationally close to the nurse, whereas the patient with a more severe need is not. Hence, consideration of need severity should trump relational proximity in situations where there is unambiguous inequality in needs.

But this does not mean that impartial consideration or calculation of needs always should trump partiality based on relational proximity. As I said previously, unequal needs are also represented by needs that are too different to be compared (i.e. the needs are unequal, but of equal moral relevance). In those cases it is not obvious which needs should be prioritised. Consider again the district nurse helping a patient with the morning toileting. According to her schedule, she knows she is running out of time. Fifteen minutes away is another patient waiting for her to facilitate breakfast. These two patients' needs are unequal and too different to be compared, but they might still be of equal moral importance (at least from the patients' perspectives). There is also unequal relational proximity in this case.

To illustrate my point further, recall the example of Tom's dilemma. If Mary's needs are unequal to the needs of the patient waiting for the room, Tom might be permitted to be partial to Mary (due to relational proximity). This is the case if – and only if – needs either are different, but of equal moral relevance, or their needs are too different to be compared, but of equal moral relevance and worth.

Their needs may be too different to be compared adequately, but still be considered as equal with regard to moral or professional relevance. Then these needs are unequal, but of equal moral relevance and worth. This means there is no qualitative difference between the needs. For instance, Mary's needs for communication, for a prolonged stay, etc., are *equal* (i.e. identical) to that of the other patient if and only if that patient's needs are more or less exactly the same. But that sameness is not very likely. Instead, their needs might be qualitatively unequal, but of equal moral relevance. If, say, the other patient's need for nursing home admission is based on decreased self-care, his or her need (i.e. the objective 'need for nursing home care') is equal to that of Mary. But there might be different reasons for needing nursing home care. This is why a patient's subjective needs also must be taken into account even when it complicates the picture.

Since relational proximity should be prioritised in situations where there is unequal relational proximity and the needs are unequal in a non-morally relevant way (not as in the 'severity of need' cases, where severity of needs should be prioritised), it follows that Tom is *permitted* to be partial towards Mary. But this is only so when Mary's needs and those of the other patient are unequal in a non-morally relevant way. In other words, the needs of nursing home care may be considered equal at an institutional level. But at the clinical level, where nursing care takes place, the needs may be considered qualitatively unequal, but of equal moral relevance. This is also why it is important to acknowledge that even though needs may be objectively equal, or unequal with equal moral relevance, they may be subjectively very distinct. For instance, from an objective point of view, if both Mary and the other patient have equal need of nursing home care, they may very well have subjectively different needs for it. And the consequences for these two individuals might be very different. Partiality must always be balanced with impartial concerns of other patients with legitimate claims for care.

So far I have only discussed cases where there is unequal relational proximity combined either with equality of need or inequality of need. Three conclusions are drawn: (1) even though a principle of relational proximity might be justified as a principle for differential treatment, severity of needs must always be a decisive element in priority decisions; (2) partiality (as giving priority to relational proximity) is permissible in cases where there is equality in needs, i.e. when needs are identical; and (3) partiality is justified when there are unequal needs that are too different to be compared, but taken to be equal in morally relevant ways. In the next subsection I will discuss cases where there is equal proximity.

Equal cases should be treated equally: cases of equality in relational proximity

The second possible implication of applying 'relational proximity' as a criterion for distributive justice is the case where there is equality in relational proximity.

The three conclusions from the previous subsection also reflect on this implication. For starters, since severity of needs always must trump, it is beside the point whether there is inequality or equality in relational proximity. As I argued above, one cannot appeal to a principle of relational proximity in acute and critical situations. Relational proximity can never in normatively significant ways override severity of needs. Hence, conclusion (1) above is valid in any such case.

But what about conclusions (2) and (3)? One may say that one can hardly be partial towards two (or more) patients at the same time. Therefore, the normative statement 'to each according to proximity' does not seem to make any sense when there is equal proximity. Still, it should not be rejected without further reflection. This is so because a nurse is often committed to more than one nursing project at the same time.

What does relational proximity amount to when two or more patients are in the same ward and the nurse is responsible for both or all of them? There is no clear-cut way of determining limits and degrees of relational proximity in such situations. I shall return to this problem in the next subsection.

For now, consider a nurse's responsibility for more than one patient in a hospital ward or in a nursing home. Partiality (i.e. the differential treatment in question) may imply that the nurse should spend more time with one patient than another. But this does not rule out the possibility of partiality towards two or more patients. For instance, parental partiality does not mean that a parent should be partial to the needs of only one of their children. And the same goes for professional partiality. Hence, the normative statement 'each according to relational proximity' makes sense even when there is equality in relational proximity. This is so when scarcity of resources makes it possible to provide proper care to only one or a few patients for whom the nurse has direct responsibility (Nordhaug and Nortvedt, 2011). A moral dilemma then arises between competing equal professional commitments.

Let me briefly mention an approach inspired by Goodin's theory of responsibility (Goodin, 1985). From Goodin's analysis of vulnerability, at least two considerations must come into play in such situations. The relative vulnerability of each patient to the professional must be taken into account in allocating responsibilities. In health care, one first has to determine how strongly a patient's need would be affected by alternative choices of action. One important question then is whether the patient can be taken care of by other nurses.

Indeed, one should always consider how strongly the patient's needs will be affected by alternative actions and choices. But how such an assessment can solve a dilemma is not clear. And the other consideration appears even less promising. It can be taken to indicate, for instance, that patients' needs should be cared for at the most cost-effective level, by personnel with less competence, or personnel with other kinds of competences. Perhaps, in some particular cases, this is the right thing to do. But it may also lead to patients being shuttlecocked in the health care system. It may also threaten the jurisdiction of some health care professions if lack of resources and claims of efficiency are the only factors when deciding which professions should take care of a patient's need.

Goodin's account might serve as a useful analytical tool for priority decision-making at a clinical level, but as argued above, the problems of prioritisation cannot be resolved at a clinical level. Moreover, even though some of these problems might be reduced by organisational structures and decisions at a higher level, they will still arise. There will always be situations where it is not evident how to prioritise between patients and between needs. And there will always be, though hopefully less often, situations where there are not enough resources to take care of all who have a legitimate claim for nursing care. Moral dilemmas of this kind are the topic of the next section.

To summarise briefly so far, we can say that partiality based on proximity might be permissible when there is equal or unequal relational proximity, if, and only if, needs are equal in a morally relevant way. But due to situational constraints, instances like these represent moral dilemmas. Several conclusions can now be drawn from this:

Unequal cases should be treated unequally (partiality–impartiality conflicts)

a   Partiality is permissible when there is unequal relational proximity and identical needs.

b   Partiality is permissible when there is unequal relational proximity and unequal needs that are relevantly equal with regard to severity and urgency (i.e. of equal moral relevance).

c   Partiality is *not* permissible when there is unequal relational proximity and needs that are unequal with regard to severity and urgency. In these cases severity and urgency of needs trump proximity.

Equal cases should be treated equally (partiality–partiality conflicts)

d   Partiality is *not* permissible when there is equal relational proximity and needs that are unequal with regard to severity and urgency. In these cases, severity and urgency of needs trump proximity.

e   Partiality is permissible when there is equal relational proximity and identical needs.

f   Partiality is permissible when there is equal relational proximity and unequal needs that are relevantly equal with regard to severity and urgency (i.e. of equal moral relevance).

Since it is extremely doubtful that human needs can ever be identical, both (a) and (e) must be considered merely hypothetical. This leaves us with the conclusion that partiality might be permissible in situations where needs may be too different to be compared in exact terms, but are still of equal moral relevance. In such cases, a nurse is permitted to be partial to the patient whom she is committed to in a nursing project.

These arguments are all consistent with distributive justice as understood from the formal principle of justice. However, this does not mean that any six of them represent simple or airtight solutions to clinical priority decisions. Besides, any such decision must be based on contextual sensitivity as well as with concern for the role-relative restriction against causing harm to patients. And, as emphasised, we are still left with certain moral dilemmas.

Partiality, tragic choices, and moral blamelessness

In the previous section some situational limits to permissible partiality were discussed and set against the formal principle of justice. In particular, the severity of needs must always be taken into account in priority decisions, and partiality based on relational proximity cannot trump severity of needs. Consequently, so far I have only said that partiality is permissible under some conditions. But under the very same conditions some unavoidable dilemmas appear. What I have in mind here are situations of equal relational proximity, i.e. situations like (e) and (f). That is, situations where there is either equality in needs or needs that are qualitatively unequal but of equal moral relevance. My goal in this section is to illustrate that since partiality as understood here represents morally desirable actions, a nurse performing such an action does something morally right and is thereby praiseworthy for doing so. If so, partiality has a normative significance that does not amount to a partial *duty* or *obligation*, but has nevertheless stronger normative connotations than a notion of *permissible* partiality. There is no suggestion here that such an argument will eliminate the portrayed moral dilemmas. I am more inclined to think that there are some implications for how we comprehend the portrayed moral dilemmas if permissible partiality is considered morally desirable under the conditions mentioned in the beginning of this chapter. In what follows, I will first discuss partiality in light of Nomy Arpaly's (2003; 2006) notion of moral desirability and praiseworthiness. Then I will address the issue of moral dilemmas and tragic choices before I make some final remarks about moral blamelessness.

Partiality, moral desirability, and praiseworthiness

According to Arpaly,

> an action is desirable if it ought to be performed (or to the extent that it would be better to perform it), and it can be desirable for moral reasons, for prudential reasons, for aesthetic reasons, or any other kind of reason.
> (Arpaly, 2006, pp. 9–10)

Arpaly makes do with intuitive assumptions, here, namely by trusting that the reason for the rightness of an action will be the same as the reason for the action: 'an action is right because it alleviates the suffering of a person, and an agent performs it in order to alleviate the suffering of a person' (Arpaly, 2003, p. 72).

It seems fair to say that a patient's need for nursing care is a *moral* appeal for nursing care. It seems reasonable to argue that the comprehension of a patient's nursing care needs is a comprehension of moral reasons, and, subsequently, that acting from the comprehension of these particular needs is to act from those moral reasons. The actions in question necessitate 'giving proper and individual care', and are matters of professional moral concern for *the particular patient for whom one has responsibility*. In some situations, these actions require the adequate and individualised performance of some degree of partiality. Hence, in those situations, partiality represents a morally desirable action for a moral reason (but also for an instrumental professional reason). Partiality based on relational proximity might therefore be important for responding to and acting on a moral reason.

When an agent performs a morally desirable action, the agent is generally entitled to praise for the action (Arpaly, 2006). According to Arpaly, an agent is morally praiseworthy if

> doing the right thing is for her to have done the right thing for the relevant moral reasons – that is, for the reasons for which the action is right (the *right reasons* clause); and an agent is more praiseworthy, other things being equal, the deeper the moral concern that has led to her action (the *concern* clause). Moral concern is to be understood as concern for what is

in fact morally relevant and not as concern for what the agent takes to be morally relevant.

(Arpaly, 2003, p. 84)

Here, 'the right reason clause' pertains to reasons for which partiality is right. In an agent-neutral sense, one might say that partiality is right because it has desirable consequences.[5] These desirable consequences relate to the common good implemented in the four main responsibilities of the nursing profession. Elsewhere I have argued that partiality is permissible under certain conditions, and is even morally desirable for moral reasons. In this sense, the reason why partiality is morally desirable is also the reason why partiality is right.

For this reason, if an act of partiality is a morally desirable act, then acting according to partiality makes the nurse praiseworthy. But it will also imply that nurses can be morally praiseworthy for doing a right action (partiality) which at the same time implies the possibility of doing something wrong (indirectly, as a consequence of the right action). Consider Tom's dilemma with regard to unequal relational proximity. From the discussion in the previous sections, we could say that Tom is permitted to be partial to Mary but not to the unknown patient waiting for the room. The same is true in dilemmas of equality in proximity. Tom is permitted to be partial to Mary and the other patients in the ward. And he is permitted to be partial to all of them for the same reasons, provided their needs are equal in a morally relevant sense. But as we have seen, the problem is that Tom, due to *situational constraints*, cannot discharge his professional commitment to provide adequate and individualised nursing care to all of these patients at the same time. As we recall from the example, 'Tom did also have to give less priority to the morning toileting of the frailest patients, and two of the patients had to stay in bed in order for him to provide a minimum of nursing care for all patients in the ward.' Again, permissible partiality might have some – more or less serious – implications for other patients. To put it another way, a morally desirable action (partiality) implies indirectly doing something wrong.[6] Partiality might not only be permissible, but also morally desirable. And the nurse who performs a morally desirable action, i.e. permissible partiality, is praiseworthy for doing so even if this implies indirectly doing something wrong. Later in this chapter, however, I will argue that this should be considered as blameless 'wrongdoing'.

Now, Arpaly's 'concern clause' indicates that praiseworthiness is *relative* to the moral concern. The more moral concern it takes to perform a certain action, the more praiseworthy the agent is for taking it (Arpaly, 2003). Arpaly takes moral concern to be a form of desire:

> To say that a person acts out of moral concern is to say that a person acts out of an intrinsic (noninstrumental) desire to follow (that which in fact is) morality, or a noninstrumental desire to take the course of action that has those features that make actions morally right.

(Arpaly, 2003, p. 84)

It is important to note that Arpaly emphasises a distinction between acting *for* reasons believed or known to be such, and acting *from* what is moral reason. Moral worth, Arpaly says, is 'fundamentally about acting for moral reasons, not about acting for reasons believed or known to be such, and distinguishing the two is important in evaluating moral agents' (Arpaly, 2003, p. 73).[7]

For an action to be morally desirable *and* of positive moral worth, and *thereby* a morally praiseworthy action, it must be done for moral reasons. Note here that there is a distinction between moral desirability and moral worth:

> Two actions that are equal in moral desirability may be of different moral worth. To give a simple example, two people may donate equal amounts of money to Oxfam, but one of them may do so out of concern for improving the state of the world, while the other does so purely at the urging of her accountant. Even if the two agents' charitable actions are equally morally desirable – both of them have done the right thing – it is not true that both agents deserves the same degree of praise.
>
> (Arpaly, 2003, p. 69)

From Arpaly's account we could say that partiality is not of moral worth if not done for the relevant moral reasons. As long as partiality has those features that make it morally right, we might say that a nurse acts out of concern if her actions are based on a desire to act from the reasons that make partiality right.

Once we have established both the 'right reason clause' and the 'concern clause' for partiality, we can say that partiality is a morally praiseworthy action. Another important aspect of moral concern is related to the problem of guilt. As Arpaly notes, doing something wrong is painful, it makes one feel guilty (2006).

This can also be formulated the other way around. That is, the morally concerned person, other things being equal, will find the thought of *not being able to do the right thing* quite painful. Hence, a nurse being concerned when confronted with a patient and his needs will find it painful not to be able to provide proper and individualised care for this patient, to not be able to perform the right action. This is in part why I will regard the moral dilemmas in health care priorities as dilemmas of a tragic nature. I will soon turn to this.

Finally, although the concern clause according to Arpaly is relative, I do not think it takes *greater* moral concern to perform an action of partiality, and that therefore nurses should be *more* praiseworthy for doing that rather than acting impartially. I think it suffices to say that nurses can be praiseworthy for actions of partiality. But in situations where the nurse has to decide which of several desirable actions of partiality to prioritise, it seems that praiseworthiness implies the possibility of doing something wrong, i.e. not providing adequate nursing care. But it might also refer to the unavoidable (and undesirable) consequences partiality has for other patients. This predicament of partiality conflicts reveals the moral dilemmas inherent in these situations.

Moral dilemmas and tragic choices

Let me start this section with a clarification: Most frequently, the notions of 'tragic choices' and 'tragic dilemmas' refer to choices and dilemmas where life is at stake and the consequences for the involved parties (including the agent) are catastrophic. One may therefore object to my application of the notion of 'tragedy' here. Moral dilemmas or difficult choices as regards patients' nursing care needs are not of a tragic nature, one may say. These are seldom about life-or-death decisions or situations that would have catastrophic results. My claim is rather that the basic and even the so-called minor needs of nursing care may very well be of fundamental importance for the patient. Since the small, daily choices concern a particular individual's life, daily priority decisions should be based on a respectful acknowledgement of these minor tragedies for the persons involved. Who am I to express how it feels to lie helpless in my bed with a wet diaper and have my morning toileting postponed, to not be comforted when I am lonely and anxious about going back home, to not receive help eating nor adequate information about my medical condition, and who am I to express how it feels to die alone in a hospital bed? And how does it feel to be the one who must postpone the morning toileting of a helpless patient, must send a lonely and anxious patient back home, or does not have the time to help a patient with their basic needs? How does it feel to know that a patient is dying alone in a hospital bed while you are busy because of resource constraints? Who am I to say that these are not minor tragedies for the persons involved? This is probably a radical way to conceive of tragedies, but I do not think it is a misconstruction.

The required mechanisms of priority in health care inevitably entail saying yes to someone with a legitimate need at the expense of someone else with an equally sound need (Ruyter et al., 2014). Saying 'no' to someone or something has to be based on sound judgment. But moral dilemmas represent cases where two claims are equally strong. Methodological approaches such as generating and refining political and clinical guidelines cannot fully capture the tragic dimension of moral dilemmas in health care prioritising. But as I have said previously, even if health care institutions made more room for partiality, and thereby reduced the problem of partial–impartial conflicts, we are still left with partial–partial dilemmas. And these are moral dilemmas of a tragic nature. This is because a tragedy is irresolvable by nature. It is irresolvable because no matter which of the available choices you decide to act on, you will inevitably do something wrong. According to Solbakk, tragedy – in an Aristotelian frame – deals with conflicts of a seemingly irresolvable nature, i.e. conflicts where the 'possibilities of a resolution in terms of "compromise" or "mediation" between the parties involved seem to represent non-existing options' (Solbakk, 2004, pp. 105–106).

Whether a moral dilemma portrays a tragic choice partly depends on the consequences of the choice. A tragic choice always leaves a moral residue and involves some degree of guilt, regret, or remorse. One cannot make a moral judgment by tossing a coin, thinking this will remove any worries or anxiety about the judgment. The result of tossing a coin isn't unimportant; indifference is not an option because tragic dilemmas involve emotional responses as well. Hence, in tragic dilemmas the nurse is under what Solbakk refers to as a '*double* constraint: the necessity to decide, amidst the absence of the possibility of making a decision not contaminated with some sort of error or guilt (*hamartia)*' (Solbakk, 2006, p. 147).[8]

According to Williams, one consequence of having to make a choice in a moral dilemma is the person's willingness to make it up to anyone who is injured by that particular choice (Williams, 1973). When it is necessary to not act on one choice, there may be 'room for nothing but regret' (Williams, 1973, p. 172). On regret, Williams says:

> These states of mind do not depend, it seems to me, on whether I am convinced that in the choice I made I acted for the best; I can be convinced of this, yet have these regrets, ineffectual or possibly effective, for what I did not do.
>
> (Williams, 1973, p. 172)

What seems paradoxical is that, in tragic dilemmas, the whole notion of 'acting for the best' loses its meaning. No matter what one chooses to do, one could not have made a better choice, simply because there is no better option available. Marcus's view that there are circumstances where the moral agent will be guilty no matter what is radical and controversial:

> Where moral conflicts occurs, there is a genuine sense in which both what is done and what fails to be done are, before the actual choice among irreconcilable alternatives, within the agent's range of options. 'You are damned if you do and you are damned if you don't.'
>
> (Marcus, 1980, p. 127)

Foot (2002) on the other hand, disputes this view, arguing that no one can be said to *be* guilty even though they might *feel* guilty after making a difficult moral choice. I think Foot is correct in her claim. Consider Tom again. There is no way out of his partial–partial dilemma; no compromise is possible, and no matter what choice he makes the result is something morally undesirable and will cause some suffering for a patient, and for himself. One's failure to make the first choice can never be compensated for by having made the other (Dancy, 1993). It is worth noting that feelings of guilt and regret come in degrees according to, I assume, what is at stake in the situation, and the implications for the patients in question. But I have already said that if partiality is a morally desirable action, and an action of moral worth, the nurse is praiseworthy. But even then, the nurse might have a feeling of regret or a feeling of guilt. But this, as will be shown below, does not mean that the nurse in fact can *be* guilty.

Tragic dilemmas and blameworthiness

Earlier in this chapter it became evident that moral concern is a decisive element in morally praiseworthy actions. One does not deserve praise for a morally desirable action if it is not done for the very same reasons that make the action right. I argued that a nurse acting partially should be praiseworthy if partiality was a morally desirable action. Partiality is justified if done for the moral as well as professional reasons that make the action right. I also said that in partial–partial conflicts, the praiseworthiness of partial actions bears an element of guilt or regret. This is what I referred to as moral dilemmas of a tragic nature. In the following, I will first present a short note on tragic dilemmas in light of Arpaly's notion of blameworthiness.

According to Arpaly, an agent is 'blameworthy for taking a morally wrong course of action out of lack of good will or out of ill will' (Arpaly, 2006, p. 15). The notion of 'will' can be taken to denote something very similar to moral concern. As Arpaly says,

> the person who does the right thing out of responsiveness to moral reasons does it out of *good will*, the person who does the wrong thing or fails to do the right thing out of a failure to respond to pertinent moral reasons displays *lack of good will* (or *moral indifference*), and the person who does the wrong thing or fails to do the right thing for the very reasons that make his course of action wrong displays *ill will*.
>
> (Arpaly, 2006, pp. 14–15)

Consider again Tom's tragic dilemma of partial–partial conflict. A single partial act, such as being partial either to Mary or to another patient on the ward, is done out of good will in so far as it is done for a moral concern for the reason that makes the action right. The problem is, as we have seen, that he *indirectly* does something morally wrong by not being able to perform another partial act of equal value. But he cannot be said to actually *do* something wrong. If Tom is blameworthy, according to Arpaly's position, it must be the case that he *fails to do the right* thing. Additionally, one is only blameworthy for a morally wrong course of action if done either out of ill will or out of lack of good will. Ill will here is defined by 'the very reasons that make his course of action wrong' (Arpaly, 2006, p. 15). This can hardly be so in Tom's case or in any partial–partial dilemma. This presupposes that partiality is the right thing to do and that the reason for partiality is what makes partiality the right thing to do. Hence, one displays ill will if one fails to act partially by taking a(nother) course of action for a reason that makes this other action *wrong*. But in partial–partial conflicts being partial does not mean one fails to be partial towards another (taking another course of action) for the reason that makes this wrong (since partiality is right).

Considering lack of good will or moral indifference, Tom has done nothing wrong per se. According to Arpaly's position, Tom displays moral indifference only in so far as he fails to do the right thing out of a *failure* to respond to moral reasons. He may respond to the moral reason to provide nursing care to his patients. His problem is that he is not *able* – due to situational constraints – to *act* according to this reason.

According to Arpaly, blameworthiness, like praiseworthiness, comes in degrees: 'other things being equal, a person is *more* blameworthy for a given course of action if she acts out of ill will than if she merely acts out of lack of good will', and 'an agent is more blameworthy for a given bad course of action the greater failure of good will she demonstrates in taking it, or, if applicable, the more ill will she demonstrates in taking it' (Arpaly, 2006, p. 15). But Arpaly also emphasises that one needs the ability to act for specific reasons, and that some circumstances make it harder or easier to do what one should do, and

> thus change the amount of good will that it takes to do the right thing or the amount of ill will or depth of indifference required to do the right thing, and thus change the amount of blame that person merits for a bad course of action.
>
> (Arpaly, 2006, p. 15)

I have argued that one cannot be blameworthy for not being able to be partial in partial–partial conflicts. That is, one cannot be blameworthy for not being able to discharge one's professional commitment to provide adequate and individualised nursing care in these kinds of conflict situations. In these dilemmas, the 'ought' of being partial does not imply a 'can' as long as a situational constraint is what makes the 'ought' impossible. Tragic dilemmas are unsolvable. And the agent is not blameworthy for indirectly doing something wrong as long as this is a result of doing something right.

Another, related argument for blamelessness is presented in Derek Parfit's book *Reasons and Persons* from 1984 (Parfit, 1984). In his discussion of consequentialism and agent-relativity, Parfit worked out the notion of blameless wrongdoing. Parfit's position has been criticised by Jonathan Dancy, who claims that consequentialism cannot account for agent-relativity. Then, in 1995, Torbjörn Tännsjö argued against Dancy to support the conclusions drawn by Parfit. I shall not take up these discussions here, but instead rely on Tännsjö's conclusions that consequentialists may argue that: 'in paying special attention to our own kin, for example, rather than to strangers, we act on consequentially approved motives while performing wrong actions – no blame, or at least diminished blame on us, then' (Tännsjö, 1995, p. 127).

The point of relevance here is that blameless wrongdoing occurs when an agent acts from his or her best set of motives, but the consequences of the action are somehow wrong. Tännsjö calls a set of motives a character: 'A character may be characterized by a specification of what actions it gives rise to (in various different situations)' (Tännsjö, 1995, p. 122) A nurse acting from the motives that guide the profession, i.e. providing adequate nursing care to individual patients, behaves according to the best set of motives available to him or her *as a nurse*. But in some situations making choices based on the best set of motives implies doing something wrong, directly or indirectly. If and when doing something wrong is a result of acting from one's best set of motives, this should be considered as blameless wrongdoing.

Concluding remarks

This chapter began with the idea of a prerogative for permissible partiality in nursing care. In this chapter I aimed to assess in which situations partiality should be permissible and in which situations it should not. Nurses are obligated by impartial considerations such as equal concerns for all patients with a legitimate need for nursing care. But as shown in the Introduction to this book, recent research indicates an imbalance between concern for the individual (partiality) and concern for all with a legitimate claim for nursing care (impartiality). Hence, it is important to investigate both situational and principle constraints to permissible partiality. The analysis was implemented by the use of the formal principle of justice. When applying 'relational proximity' as a material principle, combined with the concept of 'need', six possible conditions were identified. In situations where there is obvious inequality as regards severity of needs, the most urgent and severe needs should be decisive. But in cases where there are equally relevant needs, partiality based on relational proximity can be decisive in situations where there is inequality in relational proximity.

I also argued that as long as partiality is exercised for the right reasons and out of moral concern, it is a morally desirable action, and the nurse is praiseworthy for the action. But even though partiality can be shown to be permissible and desirable in such situations, it might have adverse consequences for other patients. In such cases, the nurse also is praiseworthy when indirectly doing something wrong that is, nonetheless, the unavoidable (and undesirable) consequences of partiality for other patients. This is the case of partial–partial conflicts, which always involve unintended negative consequences. Such difficult situations could and should be *reduced* by institutional and organisational adaptations and decisions at a macro level. Nevertheless, this is no simple or clear-cut solution. Difficult priority decisions would still exist. In particular, in situations where there is equality in relational proximity, and needs are equally relevant, the nurse is confronted with moral dilemmas of a tragic nature and feels regret, guilt, or remorse as a consequence. But as long as partiality qualifies as a desirable act of moral worth, and is permissible according to the predefined criteria, the nurse should not be blamed for being partial.

The moral dilemmas, and the difficult, sometimes even tragic, ethical choices discussed in this book concern clinical prioritisation. Partiality and clinical priority decisions are not the only ethical issues that arise in nursing care. Still, the issue of partiality influences the way we conceive of nurses' responsibility to individual patients as well as to the public. In the next and final chapter I examine how this subject can be incorporated into nursing ethics more generally.

Notes

1 Unless otherwise specified, I refer to these needs simply as 'needs'.
2 Even though such a balance might be established for certain situations, this does not mean that a balance is able to resolve conflict between partiality and impartiality in all situations.
3 The role-relative restriction against harming must also be taken into account.
4 That is, as long as the other patient isn't harmed by having his or her needs neglected or severely compromised.
5 Note that here I am only concerned about partial actions that are permissible under the conditions set at the beginning of this chapter
6 This 'wrongdoing' does not imply that patients have their needs totally neglected or are harmed in any significant way.
7 Arpaly speaks interchangeably of 'a morally praiseworthy action' and 'an action with positive moral worth' (2003, p. 69).
8 What we have here is not situations of error, which is to say that the nurse has not done anything directly wrong like inflicting pain on a patient. But it seems reasonable to say that not being able to do (another) right thing is 'contaminated' with some sort of guilt. I find this claim reasonable as long as the nurse identifies herself with the values and ideals of the professions (recall the discussion in Chapter 2).

References

Arpaly, N., 2003. *Unprincipled virtue: An inquiry into moral agency.* Oxford: Oxford University Press.

Arpaly, N., 2006. *Merit, meaning, and human bondage: An essay on free will.* Princeton, NJ: Princeton University Press.

Chappell, T., 2009. *Ethics and experience: Life beyond moral theory.* Durham, NC: Acumen.

Dancy, J., 1993. *Moral reasons.* Oxford: Blackwell.

Feinberg, J., 1973. *Social philosophy.* Englewood Cliffs, NJ: Prentice Hall.

Foot, P., 2002. *Moral dilemmas and other topics in moral philosophy.* s. 1. Oxford: Oxford University Press.

Goodin, R., 1985. *Protecting the vulnerable: A reanalysis of our social responsibilities.* Chicago: University of Chicago Press.

Marcus, R., 1980. Moral dilemmas and consistency. *Journal of Philosophy*, 77(3), pp. 121–136.

Nordhaug, M. and Nortvedt, P., 2011. Justice and proximity: Problems for an ethics of care. *Health Care Analysis*, 19, pp. 3–14.

Parfit, D., 1984. *Reasons and persons.* Oxford: Clarendon Press.

Ruyter, K., Førde, R. and Solbakk, J., 2014. *Medisinsk og helsefaglig etikk*. 3rd edn. Oslo: Gyldendal Akademisk. [Norwegian].

Solbakk, J. H., 2004. Therapeutic doubt and moral dialogue. *Journal of Medicine and Philosophy*, 29(1), pp. 93–118.

Solbakk, J. H., 2006. Catharisis and moral therapy II: An Aristotelian account. *Medicine, Health Care and Philosophy*, 9(2), pp. 141–153.

Tännsjö, T., 1995. Blameless wrongdoing. *Ethics*, 106(1), pp. 120–127.

Williams, B., 1973. *Problems of the self*. Cambridge: Cambridge University Press.

7   Towards an ethics of nursing care

In this final chapter I will explore how a framework for normative nursing ethics could incorporate a notion of permissible partiality and its principled impartial restrictions outlined in this book. More specifically, I will outline which concerns an ethics of nursing care should entail in balancing partialist and impartialist concerns. The theoretical reference for this discussion is based on Chappell's (2009) arguments for non-systematic ethical outlooks. The rationale behind this reference choice is that Chappell's emphasis on moderate particularism and his critique of systematic moral theories offer up plausible ethical guidelines for professionals. Moreover, his position is an interesting theoretical reference since nursing ethics takes place within a hybrid of impartial moral concerns and partial moral concerns. A broader ethical outlook that challenges the traditional systematic ethical theories is more sympathetic to relational and partialist concerns. However, as will be evident, the challenge is to incorporate the particular normative concerns of professional role obligations into such a *non-systematic* ethical outlook.

Chappell's defines ethics as 'the use of reason to answer the worldview-shaping question: "How should life be lived?"' (Chappell, 2009, p. 3). His question is how reason applies to this Socratic question, and he then examines how moral theories might guide us. His general conclusion is that systematic moral theory is ill fitted for providing us with the *sort of use of reason* we need for answering the question. Instead, he suggests the idea of a non-systematic ethical outlook. An ethical outlook, according to Chappell, consists of views and commitments that must be held sincerely and passionately. Besides, it must be 'as considered, rationally defensible and coherent as possible' (Chappell, 2009, p. 195). And, as maintained by Chappell,

> We want our ethical outlook to be something that can be the source of our reasons to act (*motivation*), and that can structure our real-time thinking and deciding about how to act (*deliberation*). We also want our ethical outlook to be something that, offline, can articulate and deepen our understanding of what counts as good or bad and right or wrong action, and why (*explanation*). And we want it to be something that can explain what will or would be good or bad and right or wrong action, in

future or hypothetical situations that we ourselves have not actually met, but which we or others might conceivably meet (*prediction*).

(Chappell, 2009, p. 203)

In what follows, I discuss these requirements of an ethical outlook with regard to nursing ethics as a balance between distributivist and partialist concerns.

Four requirements of a non-systematic ethical outlook

According to Chappell, four of the requirements of a non-systematic ethical outlook are motivation, deliberation, explanation, and prediction. In general, I concur with his scepticism on the prospects of systematic moral theories as exhaustive normative guidelines, but we also need to consider two weak points in Chappell's alternative position.

Chappell's position falls short regarding important differences in those obligations and responsibilities we have has private persons and those we have as professionals. Chappell can be taken either to deny the existence of such differences, or he can be taken to accept them, while regarding them as unimportant. More still, Chappell seems to be presenting an indistinct relationship between empirical statements and normativity. I shall revisit both of these critiques of Chappell's position in this chapter. But let me start with a comment on the matter of personal ethics versus professional ethics. Important for the case in point here, is Chappell's account of professional ethics:

Ethics is about what I should do *as a human being*. And it is about how my commitments under that most general description of me relate to my commitments under other, less general, descriptions. This helps to show what the various sorts of enquiries that go under the name of 'professional ethics' are all about.

(Chappell, 2009, p. 7)

From this it seems that Chappell takes one ethical outlook to guide the whole of our lives independently of the roles and positions we possess and commit to. I will bring up one problem with such an account for professional ethics. Chappell's outlook seems to be agent-relative. In other words, it is neither generalised nor universalised, but personalised (and thereby presumed to be held sincerely and passionately). As we shall see, this is a problem throughout Chappell's position. Systematic moral theories, on the other hand, are for the most part agent-neutral. This does not mean a total rejection of any form of agent-relativity, but systematic moral theories are traditionally oriented towards universality and agent-neutrality. Another problem with an ethical outlook that purports to incorporate all types of roles we possess is that many of these roles involve obligations that are role-relative. These obligations are often regulated by law and are externally imposed on the role-taker. They incorporate some personal comprehension of the values and ideals that inform the role, yet one cannot and should not expect them to be held passionately. The example I have in mind here is of course the role of a professional nurse. The problem, then, with Chappell's position is that very few of the ethical obligations and duties we have as private persons are of such a character. An ethical outlook that overlooks such differences is inadequate, for instance, in cases where there is a conflict between our role-obligations and our obligations as private persons.[1] In what follows, I will explore and discuss Chappell's account of the four roles that an ethical outlook should play.

Motivation

> Nobody sane normally or standardly acts so as to realize utility, or 'on the motive of duty' (Kant's own phrase), or 'for the sake of virtue' itself (Aristotle's own phrase). What really motivates most of us, most of the time, at least if we are moderately good people or better and are not being distracted by false motives such as concern about 'what others will think', is *love*.
>
> (Chappell, 2009, p. 204)

Chappell's first claim is that our ethical outlook in itself gives us reasons for action. His assertion is that love constitutes our most pervasive and deepest motivation, and thereby generates our reasons for action. Like the notion of care, love joins a list of concepts that are hard to define. Chappell's use of the notion of love should be understood in a broad sense. It includes love for those nearest and dearest, and it includes love for valued places and artworks, etc. (Chappell, 2009). Our objects of love are thus very different from each other, and they differ from person to person. And the semantics of the concept are as broad as its scope. The common denominator seems to be whom and what we care about. And I take the notion of love here to connote a wide spectrum of all we care about. We could, however, add the adjective 'deeply' to this notion. Indeed, love is stronger than simply caring about something or someone. Thus, Chappell's claim about what motivates us appears sensible: It is perfectly human to experience love as a deep motivational element. Most of us, if not all, can bring to mind occasions where love is what provided us with reason for a certain action. But such an account of motivation is not unproblematic.

The first problem arises from what appears to be indistinctness between the descriptive and the normative in Chappell's position. We should bear in mind that Chappell's point of departure is a critique of systematic moral theories for not being able to address our real-life ethical challenges and questions. As regards motivation, he says, systematic moral theories cannot in themselves be sources for our reasoning because they disregard love. In other words, they do not provide any adequate account of motivation since they deny the role of love in morality, Chappell says. Or, at best, moral theories admit a filtered form of love to be a source of motivation, where love must be subject to constraints of justice and other virtues (2009).

But within Chappell's lines of reasoning on motivation lies an ambiguity that also influences his alternative position: It is one thing to state that love *de facto* motivates us, but quite another to say that love *should* motivate us. Here I am not alluding to an 'is–ought fallacy'; it is rather a general ambiguity in Chappell's account. If Chappell's project is only a descriptive one, his account of what motivates us appears reasonable. But Chappell's account of motivation appears ambiguous about the matter of normativity. His account of a wide conception of love as reason-generating is problematic. For one, an ethical outlook is agent-relative. This implies that my ethical outlook is, or very likely is, different from your ethical outlook and the ethical outlook of other people. What motivates me does not have to be what motivates you, and vice versa. But interpersonal differences need not trouble this account.

Perhaps the most challenging issue as regards normative ambiguity relates to the fact that our reasons need not be very consistent. In particular, an intrapersonal inconsistency is problematic for an account that renders love (in a wide sense) as reason-generating. Suppose, for instance, I stop caring deeply about a certain person, and grow to dislike him instead. This change in my feelings would probably alter my motivation for doing something good for this person. But it does not follow that the change in my feelings actually removes my moral duty to do good to him. There is also a problem here concerning the direction or the objects of our love. Consider a person who cares deeply for an extreme radical conservative project and experiences a deep motivational force that seems to justify performing a terrible act. In this case the motivation does not in fact justify the behaviour. I return to the link between motivation and decision-making in the next section. At this point I only want to stress the dangerous prospect of stating that love (as an intrinsically part of our ethical outlook) is what gives us reasons for action *without* simultaneously accounting for any notion of value judgment or normative evaluation.

Admittedly, Chappell would most probably agree with these points. And he admits that love should be subject to constraints from what can be termed impartial and agent-neutral concerns in morality. But if the intention of the ethical outlook only is to describe reality (or what seems to be reality or what usually is reality), then the question is how much weight should be ascribed to impartial and agent-neutral concerns. This means that the question of normativity is unavoidable. Since the claim here is that love should be subject to impartial and agent-neutral concerns, the presupposition seems to be that it is undesirable if love isn't subject to such constraints. And if an ethical outlook is supposed to be normative (and only normative), it also has to address the issue of motivation more profoundly.

In professional ethics, this is perhaps even more important. Professional activities, such as nursing care, take place within legal frameworks and professional ethical guidelines that emphasise, for instance, equality and impartial distribution of collective goods. A conception of motivation in nursing care should articulate the difference between the merely descriptive and the normative. There is something odd about categorising motivations as good or bad, right or wrong, without any reference to context, the role, or the action to which the motivation applies. It appears, however, far easier to tell what is (definitively) bad or wrong than what is right. As for nursing care, it is not contentious to say that a nurse who is motivated by economic reward at the expense of professional values and norms, for instance, is a nurse whose behaviour is based on the wrong type of motivation. But then it is the nurse, not the motivation (i.e. economic reward) per se, who is the 'holder' of what is morally bad. Perhaps a non-systematic framework for nursing ethics cannot adequately capture anything more here than what should *not* qualify as a legitimate motivational force, or as reason-generating.

And there is also a question of how a criterion of motivation should be understood in professional contexts as well as in other role contexts. One could say that a nurse's profession entails caring deeply about nursing, or about her patients, and that this caring provides the motivation for particular nursing activities. This is not unthinkable, but still hypothetical. In the discussion of Blum's account of professional roles, in Chapter 2, I argued that one cannot expect nurses to really care deeply about every patient (or love them), nor about the values or ideals that inform one's profession. Sometimes a nurse might care deeply for a patient, for instance in long-term care where the nurses and patients grow to know each other in a more 'personal' way than in an emergency ward. But such deep caring is not the general motivational *force* in nursing care. And, as I also argued above, nursing care is (and should be) based on role-relative concerns for the patient's objective and subjective needs. Agent-relativity (in a personal sense) and subjectivity should not play a decisive role in professional care. Hence, to use the notion of love to describe concerns for patients stretches the relational value of interpersonal care too far. I will argue that love or caring deeply is a misplaced concept as regards *the* motivational force in nursing.

Since the use of love as a justification for certain decisions may lead to the arbitrary treatment of patients, we should avoid it as a normative ideal in nursing care. As for the question of partiality, I have argued that personal preferences cannot and should not justify partiality as understood here. I have argued that relational proximity to a patient is what allows the nurse to sensibly grasp the patient's situation and his or her needs, and thereby provide adequate and individualised nursing care (to carry out a nursing project). Furthermore, partiality towards the patient in some cases is what makes it possible to fulfil the nursing project. We could expect that a patient's well-being is reason enough. It is important to note that these are normative statements, premised on the view that it is the patient and his or her needs that offer justification for decisions. The motivation is therefore professional, not personal, as Chappell seems to argue, and it arises from the care receiver to whom the action is directed.

Deliberation

The second required element in an ethical outlook according to Chappell concerns decision-making. Chappell states that the ethical outlook should structure our thinking and decisions on how to act. Maybe there is nothing but an analytical distinction between reasons for action and deliberation about how to act. This point is also Chappell's departure when he argues that the shortcomings in systematic moral theories regarding motivation lead to shortcomings regarding deliberation. According to Chappell, moral theorists try to avoid this critique by emphasising that the constraint of morality concerns the form of deliberation, not the subject or content of it. Hence, Chappell's argument is that we need an ethical outlook that includes both content and form, but that moral theories cannot provide us with this. This is not a total rejection of moral theories. It is not unlikely that we sometimes make good decisions out of concern for utility, duties, or virtues. Chappell's suggestion is, however, that what motivates us is what we love (or care deeply about), and this is also what structures our deliberations. Our ethical outlook provides its own reasons for action and therefore also the content and form to our deliberations, says Chappell. But it turns out that the challenges of his account of motivation affect his account of deliberation as well. Again, the puzzle is the normative ambiguity in Chappell's position. While it seems sensible that motivation structures our deliberations, it is unclear how and why motivation based on love (or caring deeply) *should* structure our deliberations. Chappell is somewhat imprecise on this point, but this question is unavoidable even if his perspective of an ethical outlook only aims to be descriptive. The normative question is again unavoidable because it is unclear from the beginning how and to what extent love should be subject to the constraints of impartial and agent-neutral concerns. When love has been subject to such concerns (in one way or another), is it then love that structures our deliberation? Aren't we then left with a filtered (to use Chappell's term) kind of genuine motivation? If so, this must imply a filtered structure of our deliberation as well, both in content and form. And it is this 'filtering' of our deepest motivation that settles the problem for Chappell's account.

This problem becomes apparent in the face of seemingly conflicting values or ideals and uncertainty on how to deliberate. Our deepest motivations sometimes conflict with impartial and agent-neutral concerns and duties. As we have seen, this is particularly evident in professional contexts. In nursing care, deliberations about how to act must take into account impartial concerns such as fairness. Nursing ethics must be structured around different and sometimes competing normative considerations. A mere description of what in fact motivates nurses is not very helpful, nor is it useful to describe how deliberations are carried out. That is, a mere description is not effective since the aim of an ethical outlook according to Chappell's account, is to be a source of reason to act, and can structure our thinking and deliberation about how to act. Once more the general problem in Chappell's position regarding indistinctness between private life and professional roles is apparent, namely, that professional roles are subject to moral obligations that in principle affect (and should affect) deliberations.

Despite these problems there are some important insights from Chappell's perspective on professional ethics. Nursing ethics needs to be tailored to the specific issues that are endemic to nursing. From the discussion of professional role morality, we saw that nursing as a vocation is neither personal nor impersonal. Instead, an ethics of nursing care lies somewhere between these poles. To follow the analogue from Blum's discussion of roles versus vocations, nursing is not a role subjected to impersonal job descriptions, i.e. the nurse is not guided solely by impersonal or impartial moral obligations. A more personal comprehension of the values that inform nursing is essential for providing adequate and individualised nursing care. But this personal understanding does not entail subjectivism; it is not agent-relative in a deep personal sense, yet it still cannot be grasped by systematic moral theories alone. Although there are some problems in placing professional ethics under a more general 'ethical umbrella' that applies to everyday lives, as Chappell does, his critique of moral theories seems to hit the mark for professional ethics.

Deliberation is a process of weighing options in order to judge how to act in a situation at hand. Take a look at the following statement: 'It is quicker to change a sanitary pad than to bring patients to the bathroom. For this reason, they are rarely taken to the bathroom, but instead changed into a pad.'[2] This quotation from a community nurse exemplifies the concerns that inspired my engagement in the subject of this book: the hampered ability to provide adequate and individualised nursing care in the face of greater resource constraints. The quotation is an example of deliberations that are not based on a professional assessment of patients' needs. Putting a sanitary pad on a patient instead of taking him or her to the bathroom is not a result of an ethical deliberation motivated by concern for the patient's well-being, integrity, etc. Instead, it is a result of resource constraints and rigid time schedules, when one has to make choices that are second best. An important question is whether second best is good enough. And which principles can inform what is good enough in cases like these? I am concerned that impartial rules and principles cannot always help nurses make choices about how to fulfil their duties in the way that partiality can. Partiality gives room for nurses to provide full-fledged care within the constraints of institutional settings, impartial distributivist concerns, and deontological restrictions. Hence, nursing ethics should incorporate arguments for partiality. In this book I have tried to work out such arguments. Deliberations should be transparent and open to criticism, and should inform an ongoing debate on the role of partiality and impartiality in nursing care.

Explanations

One of the roles of systematic moral theories is simply to determine right actions from wrong actions. But Chappell (along with many of us, I presume) wants us to be guided by ethical outlooks that reflect the *truth* that becomes apparent in particular situations. And, not surprisingly, he argues that moral theories fail at this point as well: The tendency among moral theorists who admit that their moral theory fails to address motivation and deliberation, is to emphasise that their theory's strength lies in explaining the rightness or goodness of our motivation and deliberation (Chappell, 2009). As indicated, Chappell admits that moral theories sometimes provide satisfying answers to this issue, but not as a result of their systematic character. I shall not offer any objections to this critique. But again it is unclear in what way an agent-relative and particularistic ethical outlook à la Chappell can offer a better solution. The main obstacle here is that the critique of moral theories puts the alternative in the shade. In other words, it is hard to find an adequate *explanation* of how a non-systematic ethical outlook can address the issue of explanation. Of course, we should keep in mind that Chappell's account of a plausible ethical outlook is particularistic and agent-relative. A particularistic outlook typically allows explanations of good and bad, right and wrong to vary depending on situational circumstances. But it is not obvious how we can determine the true explanations of good and bad and right and wrong within such a perspective. But since agents have different motivations (depending on what they love or care about), and therefore deliberate differently in similar situations, where does the true explanation of right and wrong and good and bad come from, and what are the differences between them? And what role does explanation play within a particularistic outlook? Suppose you and I have completely different ethical points of view in a particular case. Since we might have different ethical outlooks we might have different opinions of what counts as the right thing to do and what counts as the wrong thing to do in this particular case. It can also be the case that you and I might agree that a certain action is right, but we might have different explanations for the rectitude of this action. These situations need not contradict the particularistic and agent-relative perspectives on ethics. But there is something odd about the claim that a particularistic and agent-neutral outlook in itself brings about *explanations of the truth*. If the truth about what is right or wrong, good or bad, is agent-relative, without any claim for consensus or 'objective truth', the whole idea about an ethical outlook as action-guiding appears strange. Hence we are left with a framework whose only function is to articulate our individual beliefs and desires. While this line of reasoning might misrepresent Chappell's usage of 'the truth', since he only seems to claim that a plausible ethical outlook aims to pursue the truth about rightness or wrongness, goodness or badness, it still raises some fundamental questions as to how 'truth' should be comprehended.

    In another usage, 'the truth' is what reflects the idea of an objective moral reality. In this sense the truth reflects a moral phenomenon of normative significance (right or wrong, good or bad), and any action based on a comprehension of this truth can obviously be explained (and justified) by reference back to this truth. Needless to say, we now are left with some delicate questions concerning particularism, agent-relativity, and moral realism. It is beyond my ambitions to address these issues in any comprehensive manner in this book.[3] Of interest here is how we can explain the rightness or wrongness of partiality in nursing care from a non-systematic ethical outlook. In nursing care, as I have argued throughout this book, impartial moral values are fundamentally important, and explanations of right and wrong and good and bad need to reflect this importance. But to be plausible in the context of nursing, the values that deeply inform the nursing profession as a relational endeavour must also be taken into account. Besides, the undertaking of these role-relative duties is particularistic in the sense that they depend on the nurse's understanding of the values that are central to nursing care in the particular situation at hand. And it is therefore also particularistic with regard to the individualities of the patients to whom the nursing activity is directed. Hence, in nursing care an explanation of the moral 'quality' of an action needs to combine impartial systematic perspectives that inform nursing, and the more particularistic role-relative concern that endorses partiality. An explanation for the moral orientation of partiality is dependent on some sort of balance between such concerns. This was the subject of discussion in Chapter 6. Again we are reminded of the problematic indistinctness between the private and the professional in Chappell's account. Although his critique of systematic moral theories appears sensible, his (vague) suggestion for a non-theoretical particularistic outlook is not easily applicable in professional contexts. Nursing ethics cannot be particularistic and agent-relative in a strict sense since it has to incorporate some principles of impartiality (such as justice as fairness, assessments of needs, and a deontological restriction against harming).

Prediction

According to Chappell (and many others), not accounting adequately for context is the main problem of prediction in systematic moral theories. To the extent that there are similar cases, moral theorists are correct in their account of prediction. However, Chappell is right that there are no qualitatively indiscernible cases. There are only cases that are more or less similar. But moral theories, he says, are overly ambitious and unrealistic regarding prediction. However, if we want our ethical outlook to facilitate prediction, then we must ask what the alternative is. Chappell's point is not that a non-systematic ethical outlook would be better at prediction. His general conclusion is rather that what we need is moral perception and moral insight instead of systematic moral theories.

It is worth pointing out that Chappell does not seem to deny that some principles and values can be transferred from one situation to another (roughly similar) situation. An ethics of nursing should incorporate some degree of prediction concerning the more principle-based part of it to prevent arbitrariness. In Chapters 5 and 6 I suggested some such principles on the matter of partiality. In Chapter 5 I argued for a prerogative of partiality, a prerogative that in turn also implied a role-relative restriction on what a nurse should be required to do to provide the best overall outcomes. I also argued for constraints on what a nurse is permitted to do. Here, a principle of not harming is a central principle. No nurse should be required or even permitted to neglect a patient's needs, even though this neglect could serve a consequentialistic norm of best overall results. Whereas Chapter 5 mainly concerned consequentialism versus partiality, Chapter 6 was oriented towards partiality and the formal principle of justice. Here, I suggested that relational proximity between a nurse and a patient, coupled with needs assessments, should work as a material principle that differentiates between equal and unequal cases. The outcome was a framework categorising partiality as permissible if there is *equality in needs in either of two forms*: Needs can be identical with regard to severity and urgency, for example, and needs can be unequal but of equal moral relevance with regard to severity and urgency. In both cases, I argued that partiality is permissible whether or not there is equality in relational proximity.

Concluding remarks

An ethics of nursing care is not only about impartial duties and systematic guidelines that are externally placed on any nurse. The role-relative ethical concerns in nursing also have to account for contextual elements such as patients' subjective needs, and nurses' own professional comprehension of values when impartial duties and guidelines are applied. Accordingly, professional ethics should balance systematic and principle-based ethics and particularistic and partial ethical concerns. Therefore, I agree with Chappell that a professional ethical outlook cannot and should not be based solely on *systematic* impartial moral theories or perspectives. I also agree that it should provide space for a more particularistic ethical perspective, including partial concerns. But when articulating his ethical outlook, Chappell does not seem to account for the complexities of professional role obligations. An unsystematic ethical outlook such as the one Chappell seems to defend has to account for the normative facts of professional ethics.

In the end, to argue for partiality is to argue for the value of individualised and adequate nursing care. But regardless of how partiality is justified, it has some inevitable consequences for the parties affected. Nurses are nevertheless faced with dilemmas that cannot be captured within a language of any such frameworks. These are what I called the minor tragedies, and they will persist regardless of whether nursing ethics is systematic or non-systematic – or something in between. Dilemmas regarding minor tragedies might have severe consequences for patients on *both* sides of the coin, and have a deep impact on the nurse regardless of the choice. One cannot necessarily predict these dilemmas. But an ethics of nursing care incorporating permissible partiality might smooth the process of coming to terms with these predicaments. And perhaps the best lesson we can learn from Chappell's anti-theoretical approach, and I would also say moderate virtue theoretical position, is that moral perception and moral sensitivity to the particular individual patient and his or her vulnerabilities are crucial. Perhaps that's the best we can hope for.

Notes

1 According to Chappell (2009) *performing* well in the different roles we occupy is also a concern about performing well in the whole of our lives. Chappell admits that there might be conflicts between certain roles we have and the way we live our lives overall, but doesn't seem to address this question any further.
2 'Det er raskere å skifte en bleie enn å forflytte folk til toalettet. Så de får ofte ikke toalettbesøk, men heller en bleie.' My translation. Norwegian Broadcasting Corporation: www.nrk.no/helse-forbruk-og-livsstil/1.8336790 Retrieved 14 January 2017.
3 See for instance Dancy (1993) and Nortvedt (2012).

References

Chappell, T., 2009. *Ethics and experience: Life beyond moral theory*. Durham, NC: Acumen.

Dancy, J., 1993. *Moral reasons*. Oxford: Blackwell.

Nortvedt, P., 2012. The normativity of clinical health care: Perspectives on moral realism. *Journal of Medicine and Philosophy*, 37(3), pp. 295–309.

Norwegian Broadcasting Corporation. www.nrk.no/helse-forbruk-og-livsstil/1.8336790 [Accessed on 14 January 2017].

Oakley, J. and Cocking, D., 2001. *Virtue ethics and professional roles*. Cambridge: Cambridge University Press.

Index